AF794194

European School of Oncology

Monographs

Series Editor: U. Veronesi

L. Denis (Ed.)

The Medical Management of Prostate Cancer

Springer-Verlag Berlin Heidelberg New York
London Paris Tokyo

Professor Dr. Louis Denis

Algemeen Ziekenhuis Middelheim
Lindendreef 1
B-2020 Antwerpen, Belgïe

The European School of Oncology gratefully acknowledges sponsorship for the Task Force received from Aktiebolaged Leo-Pharmacia Group, Helsingborg, Sweden, whose engagement in the research on prostate cancer has resulted in the origination and development of estramustine phosphate (Estracyt®) and polyestradiol phosphate (Estradurin®)

ISBN-13: 978-3-642-73240-9 e-ISBN-13: 978-3-642-73238-6
DOI: 10.1007/978-3-642-73238-6

Library of Congress Cataloging-in-Publication Data. The Medial management of prostate cancer. (Monographs / European School of Oncology) 1. Prostate–Cancer–Hormone therapy. 2. Prostate–Cancer–Chemotherapy. I. Denis, L. II. Series: Monographs (European School of Oncology) [DNLM: 1. Prostatic Neoplasms–therapy. WJ 752 M489]
RC280.P7M43 1988 616.99'463061 88-6436
ISBN-13: 978-3-642-73240-9

This work is subject to copyright. All rights are reserved, whether the whole or part of the material is concerned, specifically the rights of translation, reprinting, re-use of illustrations, recitation, broadcasting, reproduction on microfilms or in other ways, and storage in data banks. Duplication of this publication or parts thereof is only permitted under the provisions of the German Copyright Law of September 9, 1965, in its version of June 24, 1985, and a copyright fee must always be paid. Violations fall under the prosecution act of the German Copyright Law.

© Springer-Verlag Berlin Heidelberg 1988
Softcover reprint of the hardcover 1st edition 1988

The use of general descriptive names, trade names, trade marks, etc. in this publication, even if the former are not especially identified, is not to be taken as a sign that such names, as understood by the Trade Marks and Merchandise Marks Act, may accordingly be used freely by anyone.

Product Liability: The publisher can give no guarantee for information about drug dosage and application thereof contained in this book. In every individual case the respective user must check its accuracy by consulting other pharmaceutical literature.

Printing: Druckhaus Beltz, Hemsbach/Bergstr. Bookbinding: J. Schäffer GmbH & Co. KG, Grünstadt
2123/3145-543210

Foreword

Starting in 1986, the European School of Oncology has expanded its activities in postgraduate teaching, which consisted mainly of traditional disease-orientated courses, by promoting new educational initiatives. One of these is the cloister seminars, short meetings intended for highly qualified oncologists and dealing with specific, controversial aspects of clinical practice and research. Another is the institution of permanent study groups, also called task forces, where a limited number of leading experts are invited to meet once a year with the aim of defining the state of the art and possibly reaching a consensus on developments and treatment in specific fields of oncology.

This series of ESO Monographs was designed with the specific purpose of disseminating the results of the most interesting of the seminars and study groups, and providing concise and updated reviews of the subjects discussed.

It was decided to keep the layout very simple in order to keep costs to a minimum and make the monographs available in the shortest possible time, thus overcoming a common problem in medical literature: that of the material being outdated even before publication.

Umberto Veronesi
Chairman, Scientific Committee
European School of Oncology

Table of Contents

Introduction
L. DENIS 1

Aspects of Epidemiology, Pathogenesis and Natural History of Prostatic Cancer
F. H. SCHRÖDER 3

Oncogenes, Tumour Markers and Monoclonal Antibodies
L. ANDERSSON 9

The Endocrinological Basis for Hormonal Therapy
M. MOTTA 19

Estrogens and Estramustine Phosphate
L. ANDERSSON 37

Antiandrogens
G. H. JACOBI 43

Luteinizing Hormone Releasing Hormone Agonists
L. DENIS 49

Chemical Adrenal Blockade Treatment
L. DENIS 59

Total Androgen Blockade
F. H. SCHRÖDER 65

Second-Line Endocrine Treatment
G. H. JACOBI 73

Chemotherapy
A. T. VAN OOSTEROM 77

The Clinical and Financial Implications of Immediate or Deferred Treatment in Patients with Advanced Prostatic Cancer
P. H. SMITH 83

Treatment Recommendations for Daily Practice
S. ROCCA-ROSSETTI 93

List of Contributors

PROF. L. ANDERSSON
Department Urology, Karolinska Hospital, Box 60500, 10401 Stockholm, Sweden

PROF. L. DENIS
Department of Urology, A.Z. Middelheim, Lindendreef 1, 2020 Antwerp, Belgium

PROF. G. JACOBI
Department of Urology, Klinikum der Johannes Gutenberg-Universität, Postfach 3960, Langenbeckstrasse 1, 6500 Mainz, Federal Republic of Germany

PROF. M. MOTTA
Department of Physiology, Istituto di Endocrinologia, Universita di Milano, via A. del Sarto 21, 20129 Milano, Italy

PROF. S. ROCCA-ROSSETTI
Clinica Urologica, Universitá di Torino, Ospedale Maggiore S. Giovanni Battista, Corso Polonia 14, 10100 Torino, Italy

PROF. F. SCHRÖDER
Department of Urology, Erasmus University Hospital, Dr. Molenwaterplein 40, 3015 GD Rotterdam, The Netherlands

MR. P.H. SMITH
Department of Urology, St. James's University Hospital, Beckett Street, Leeds LS9 7TF, Great Britain

PROF. A.T. VAN OOSTEROM
Department of Oncology, Universitair Ziekenhuis Antwerpen, Wilrijkstraat 10, 2520 Edegem, Belgium

Introduction

L. Denis

Department of Urology, A. Z. Middelheim, Antwerp, Belgium

Cancer of the prostate is one of the most prevalent tumours in males in the industrialised world; most of these men present with metastatic disease at the time of initial diagnosis. We know that approximately 50% of these patients show objective response with androgen withdrawal,, and that subjective improvements may occur in up to 80% of the patients. However, nearly all these patients eventually relapse and are then usually unresponsive to further androgen withdrawal. The response to second-line hormonal treatment, no matter how aggressive, almost never exceeds 30%, defining advanced metastatic prostatic cancer as an incurable disease. Renewed interest in the treatment of this disease has been stimulated by the advent of new drugs that offer the hope that they may be superior to existing therapy, whether given alone or in combination treatment. The acquisition of new research information, the development of methodology in clinical research and the proliferation of new drugs and other forms of therapy have flooded the literature to the extent that facts tend to be distorted and distortions appear to become facts for the wary physician.

The European School of Oncology requested a concise review of the medical management of prostatic cancer in the framework of its Task Force programme. In this programme a multidisciplinary team of experts on the subject meet informally to define the state of the art on a particular problem. The workshop on prostatic cancer in Venice in June 1987 led to this monograph. It is clear that the views expressed are really the end result of a broad European consensus development in which dozens of medical schools and scientific organisations have contributed to the conclusions. We have tried to acknowledge this by listing appropriate references in the text. In addition, we should like to acknowledge other scientific or technical contributions to this volume by expressing our gratitude to the following advisers and helpers: Drs. Per Hedlund, Ann Charlotte Kinn and Peter Ekman of Stockholm, Dr. G.J. van Steenbrugge of Rotterdam, Mr. Don Newling of Hull, Dr. Charles Mahler of Antwerp, Dr. Donato Randone of Turin, Dr. R. Maggi and Dr. S. Zopi of Milan for advice; Mrs. Ann Hopper of Leeds, Mrs. A. Gasparini of Milan, Mrs. Rita Denie and Mrs. Chris Ploegaert of Antwerp, and, last but not least, the secretarial team of the European School of Oncology, Mrs. Sheila McGrath, Mrs. Louise Rutledge, Mrs. Marije de Jager and Dr. Alberto Costa for their enthusiastic dedication to the project.

Mrs. Barbara Montenbruck was kind and expert enough to speed this project through the Springer edition in its present form.

Aspects of Epidemiology, Pathogenesis and Natural History of Prostatic Cancer

F. H. Schröder

Department of Urology, Erasmus University, Rotterdam, The Netherlands

Prostatic cancer is the second most frequent cause of cancer death in males in most countries of the Western world, causing 9 to 10% of all cancer deaths every year. This death rate is exceeded only by lung cancer, and is followed by deaths from gastrointestinal tumors. Incidence and death from prostatic carcinoma are strongly age dependent, 75% of all prostatic carcinomas being diagnosed between the ages of 55 and 75 years.

Many aspects of prostatic carcinoma are poorly understood. Progression as part of the natural course of the disease as well as under treatment is extremely difficult to predict. When prostatic cancer is diagnosed incidentally as focal disease which is microscopically limited to several visual fields and which is well differentiated, the risk of progression is very low. Based on figures of clinical incidence, it must be assumed that only 1 in 1,000 to 3,000 patients with an incidentally found focal tumor will progress to the clinical and metastatic state.

Even when a distinct nodular mass can be palpated within the prostate, progression to metastatic disease may not occur during the lifetime of a given patient. In spite of the fact that several parameters, such as tumor size and grade of malignancy, show strong correlations with the tendency of a given tumor population to progress, it is still clinically impossible to predict which patient's tumor will show progression and which will not.

Decisions whether to treat locally confined carcinoma have to deal with the dilemma just described. But even in patients with metastatic disease, great individual differences in the rate of progression are found. Fifty per cent of patients who undergo endocrine management for metastatic disease will progress within 2 to 3 years. Some never respond in any clinically appreciable way to hormonal management, whilst others respond for long periods and die of other causes.

The extreme variability of the clinical behaviour of this disease makes any treatment decision difficult, especially as far as localized disease is concerned. It is essential for the clinician who deals with this disease to have a good knowledge of prognostic factors and indicators for response to treatment. He will often have to apply this knowledge in daily, individual treatment decisions if he is to manage his patients with prostatic cancer properly.

Epidemiology

For a good understanding of many features of prostatic carcinoma, it is essential to be familiar with some of the terms that are used to describe prostatic carcinoma found only at post-mortem examination and incidentally in clinical specimens removed for the treatment of BPH. Tumors found at autopsy which have not led to symptoms and to the diagnosis of clinical disease during the life time of a patient are often called latent carcinomas. They are named occult if metastases are present. Prostatic carcinoma is named focal carcinoma if one or more small foci are encountered at the examination of the organ at autopsy or after surgical removal of prostatic hyperplasia for obstruction. Carcinoma of the prostate that is not evident at clinical examination by means of rectal palpation, but which is diagnosed in BPH specimens after surgical removal, is called incidental carcinoma. Incidental carcinoma may be focal or may be locally extensive. Many definitions of incidentally found focal carcinoma are available. In the recommendation of the World Health Organisation (WHO), every tumor exceeding 2 to 3 microscopic fields at a magnification of 200 times would be called locally extensive. In most clinical series incidental carcinoma is found in 8 to 12% of routine histological sections of BPH tissue and Cantrell and coworkers [1] have shown a strong prognostic correlation for tumor that occupies less or more than 5% of the slide surface available for review.

Of great scientific interest is the question of what causes progression from focal to clinically manifest metastatic disease. In some parts of the world, especially well studied is Japan, the incidence of prostatic carcinoma is 10 to 15 times lower than in most Western countries. When Japanese males migrate from Japan to Hawaii or to the United States, the incidence rises, but during the first generation does not quite reach the level found in the native Americans. Despite this, the incidence of true focal metastatic carcinoma found at autopsy or incidentally found at prostatic surgery for BPH is very similar in Japan and other Western countries. These facts indicate that factors must be present in the life style of the Western civilised world that promote the progression from focal to clinical prostatic cancer. The phenomenon can certainly not be explained on purely rational grounds. Identification of the promoting factors seems to be of great importance and might lead to preventive measures in the management of this disease. More information on this complex subject can be found in the recent publications of Akazaki [2], Breslow [3] and Zaridze [4].

Another important feature of the epidemiology of prostatic carcinoma lies in the fact that mortality rates of prostatic cancer are much lower than incidence rates in the same populations. This discrepancy is highest in the early stages. In series of patients treated by radical prostatectomy or radiotherapy with curative intention, roughly 25% of patients will die of their malignant disease. Even in the more advanced stages only 50 to 65% of patients will die of prostatic cancer. This is due to the high incidence of competing causes of death in the age groups involved and by the slow rate of progression of prostatic cancer in many individuals. This phenomenon must be seriously considered in treatment decisions, especially in older and generally less healthy patients. However, as mentioned earlier, it is still very difficult, if not impossible, to predict which patients will have long progression-free intervals. For that unfortunate reason it remains difficult to individualize therapeutic measures according to the clearly smaller risk of dying of prostatic carcinoma that some patients are retrospectively shown to have.

More complete reviews of the epidemiology of prostatic carcinoma have recently been published by Wynder [5] and Flanders [6].

Pathogenesis

From what has been said above, it is clearly evident that prostatic cancer comprises a number of sub-entities, such as focal disease, locally extensive non-metastatic disease, hormone-dependent metastatic disease and hormone-independent metastatic disease, which are associated with different morphologies and an extremely variable prognosis. Differences in incidence and prognosis between these sub-entities are so large that a different state of malignant cellular transformation must be assumed. This would indicate that at least 3 to 4 mutational steps are necessary for the development of the hormone-independent prostatic carcinoma, which determines the fate of most of our patients. At this moment it is not known what causes prostatic cancer nor is it known what causes the various steps that finally lead to a tumor with the potential to metastasize and to kill the patient.

The natural development described here is parallelled by a morphogenesis that ranges from well differentiated focal to anaplastic and widely disseminated disease. Most prostatic carcinomas arise in that area of the prostate described by McNeal [7] as the peripheral zone. As a result, most can be palpated by means of rectal examination in an early stage of development. On a microscopic level, McNeal and others described 2 early abnormalities that are probably compatible with the earliest stages of prostatic carcinoma. These consist of an abnormal budding or prostatic acini and intraductal hyperplasia which may or may not be connected with the isolated presence of a dysplastic, immature or metaplastic cell type.

In clinically manifest prostatic carcinoma tumor formations with differing architectural and cytological features are often found next to each other. These may or may not represent the development from the well to the less well differentiated state. The presence of up to 4 tumor formations with different morphological appearances may be an expression of the multifocal origin of this disease, but also points in the direction of the presence of multiple clonal populations within the same tumor. By the use of common markers, such as acid and alkaline phosphatase and prostate-specific antigen, it has been shown that morphologically different formations within the same tumor may also show different functional characteristics as far as the expression of these proteins is concerned. It seems that poorly differentiated prostatic carcinoma is more frequently associated with the hormone-independent state of this disease. Unfortunately, however, hormone independence can not reliably be predicted by any morphological characteristic so far described.

Natural History

The natural history of a disease describes its course without treatment. If one wishes to deal with the natural history of prostatic carcinoma, one has to consider separately the sub-entities mentioned above and the prognosis of the different stages of the disease at the time of clinical diagnosis. The classical article on this subject has been written by Whitmore [8].

Table 1 indicates the frequency distribution of cases of prostatic cancer within the American stage grouping A, B, C and D. It is evident that only 10 to 20% of cases are diagnosed in a locally confined state (A,B), whereas 40 to 50% are locally extensive, and 35 to 50% metastatic at diagnosis. A recent report of a large survey of the American College of Surgeons on prostatic cancer published by Mettlin et al. [9] shows a tendency towards more frequent early diagnosis.

Progression rates without treatment are not known for all stages of disease. Stage A can be subdivided into true focal disease, as defined above, and microscopically extensive disease. A study of progression rates by Cantrell [1] showed 2% progression for true focal disease and 32% progression for the microscopically more extensive disease during the follow-up period of 4 years. In the so-called focal study of the Veterans Administration Cooperative Urological Research Group (VACURG), 2 of 30 patients (6.7%) showed progression within 6.8 years without any form of treatment [10].

Very little information is available on untreated patients with locally confined nodules in the recent literature. These patients are commonly treated by radical prostatectomy or radiotherapy. The VACURG study of radical prostatectomy versus placebo, reported by Byar et al. in 1981 [10], showed progression in 7 of 20 patients (35%) in the placebo control arm within 7.7 years. This information is compatible with several other reports.

For locally extensive and metastatic prostatic carcinoma, virtually no information is available on the course of untreated disease. It was shown by Kramer et al. [11] that, independently of the extent of lymph node metastases, in N+ disease the median time to progression amounts to 80 months with no treatment. These figures are not changed significantly if radiotherapy is given or radical prostatectomy undertaken. With endocrine management the median time to progression is significantly different for locally extensive non-metastatic patients and for patients with metastatic disease.

Table 1. Frequency distribution of cases of prostatic cancer within the stages A,B,C,D

Study (reference)	Stages (%)			
	A	B	C	D
Whitmore, 1973 [8]	-	<10	40	50
McCullough, 1978 [12]	5-10	5-10	45	30-35
Catalona & Scott, 1979 [13]	< 10	15	40	35-40
VACURG & Byar, 1977 [14]	5	5	50	40

Progression rates and times to progression for untreated metastatic disease are not known.

When dealing with prostatic carcinoma, knowledge of the natural progression rates of the various stages is essential information for decision making. The risk of the disease in the stage at which it presents has to be balanced against the risk of the proposed management. Benefit in terms of improved quality of life expectancy must be seen against the background of information concerning natural history, which in this way has an impact on therapeutic decisions in this disease.

REFERENCES

1 Cantrell BB, DeKlerk DP, Eggleston JC, Boitnott JK, Walsh PC: Pathological factors that influence prognosis in stage A prostatic cancer: the influence of extent versus grade. J Urol 1981 (125):516-520
2 Akazaki K, Stemmermann GN: Comparative study of latent carcinoma of the prostate among Japanese in Japan and Hawai. JNCI 1973 (50,5):1137-1144
3 Breslow N, Chan CW, Dhom G, Drury RAB, Franks LM, Gellei B, Lee YS, Lundsberg S, Sparke B, Sternby NH, Tulinius H: Latent carcinoma of prostate at autopsy in seven areas. Int J Cancer 1977 (20):680-688
4 Zaridze DG, Boyle P, Smans M: International trends in prostatic cancer. Int J Cancer 1984 (33):223-230
5 Wynder EL, Mabuchi K, Whitmore WF: Epidemiology of cancer of the prostate. Cancer 1971 (28):344-360
6 Flanders WD: Review: prostate cancer epidemiology. The Prostate 1984 (5):621-629
7 McNeal JE: Origin and evolution of prostatic carcinoma. In: Ablin RJ (ed) Prostatic Cancer. Marcel Dekker Inc, New York/Basle 1981 pp 43-50
8 Whitmore WF: The natural history of prostatic cancer. Cancer 1973 (32):1104
9 Mettlin C, Natarajan N, Murphy GP: Recent patterns of care of prostate cancer patients in the United States: results from the surveys of the American College of Surgeons Commission on Cancer. Int Adv Surg Oncol 1982 (5):277-321
10 Byar DP, Corle DK, Veterans Administration Cooperative Urological Research Group: VACURG randomized trial of radical prostatectomy for stage I and II prostate cancer. Urology 1981 (Suppl 12,4):7-11
11 Kramer SA, Cline WA, Farnham R, Carson CC, Cox EB, Hinshaw W, Paulson DF: Prognosis of patients with stage D1 prostatic carcinoma. J Urol 1981 (125):817
12 McCullough DL: Diagnosis and staging of prostatic cancer. In: Skinner DG, deKernion JB (eds) Genito-Urinary Cancer. Saunders, Philadelpha 1978 p 295
13 Catalona WJ, Scott WW: Carcinoma of the prostate. In: Harrison JH, Gittes RF, Perlmutter AD, Stamey TA, Walsh PC (eds) Campbell's Urology. Saunders, Philadelphia 1979 p 1085
14 Byar D: VACURG studies on prostatic cancer and its treatment. In: Tannenbaum Lea M and Febger (eds) Urologic Pathology: The Prostate. New York 1977 pp 241-267

Oncogenes, Tumour Markers and Monoclonal Antibodies

Lennart Andersson

Department of Urology, Karolinska Hospital, Stockholm, Sweden

Oncogenes

Rapid progress in molecular biology and in genetic engineering in recent years has enabled the detection of changes in the genome of normal cells responsible for changes in the cell functions which may contribute to the development of cancer.

It has been known for a long time that virus infection may induce sarcoma, leukaemia or carcinoma in various animal species. Both RNA and DNA viruses may have oncogenic properties. There is evidence that viruses may be involved in the aetiology of a small number of human tumours, but the great majority of human tumours do not appear to be caused by viruses. However, investigations on the oncogenic viruses, especially the RNA viruses or retroviruses, have increased our understanding of the molecular biology of human cancer.

Two different varieties of oncogenic retroviruses exist: the slow oncogenic viruses which induce tumours after a long incubation period, and the acute oncogenic retroviruses which transform all cells if added to a cell culture, and produce tumours rapidly *in vivo* [1]. A number of acute oncogenic retroviruses have been identified and investigated. So far, acute oncogenic retroviruses have not been detected in any human tumours.

With the use of nucleic acid probes and DNA hybridization, it has been discovered that sequences of DNA, closely similar to the known virus oncogenes, are present in the normal genome of the human and of a number of animal species. These normal genes are called proto-oncogenes or cellular oncogenes [1].

DNA from human and various animal cells can be digested by restriction endonucleases and the fragments can be used to transfect cell lines in culture, that is, to combine with the DNA of those cells. It was observed that DNA from normal cells did not induce transformation of the cell line whereas DNA from tumours, human or animal, transformed the cell to proliferation in a manner similar to a malignant cell population. With modern genetic engineering techniques it has been possible to isolate the genes responsible for the transformation and to clone them. They have been found to resemble proto-oncogenes and their related virus oncogenes.

So far, 9 various oncogenes, similar to virus oncogenes, have been identified in the DNA of human tumours. The most frequently occurring oncogenes belong to the ras family. This variety of oncogenes has been found in e.g. bladder cancer, cancer of the colon and mammary cancer [2].

The conclusion must be that normal cells contain proto-oncogenes which presumably have a physiological function in the metabolism, growth and replication of the cells but do not transform the cells into a malignant behaviour. However, these proto-oncogenes may be converted to tumour oncogenes which are capable of transforming cells. It is known that activation of proto-oncogenes may occur from a variety of causes, such as a specific point mutation with alteration of their base sequence, which changes the sequence of aminoacids in the protein encoded by the gene. Chromosome translocations or rearrangements and gene amplification, in which extra copies of the proto-oncogene are inserted into the genome, may also result in the activation of proto-oncogenes.

About 20 different oncogenes have been identified. Their participation in the induction of cancer is believed to be associated with their production of proteins which are usually enzymes or hormones. Several oncogenes produce protein kinases which transfer phosphate groups to the tyrosine residues of protein. Normal cells contain very small amounts of tyrosine-phosphorylated proteins, whereas the concentration may be enhanced manyfold in cells transformed by the appropriate virus oncogenes [3]. Phosphorylation normally occurs mainly at serine and threonine sites. It has been found that several proteins are phosphorylated at tyrosine sites in cancer cells. There is evidence that phosphorylation of tyrosine may be important in the oncogene-induced development of uncontrolled cell growth [4].

Production of growth factors in tumour cells is probably a function of oncogenes. It is known that a virus oncogene of the sis-family produces a protein similar or identical to the platelet-derived growth factor [5] and another oncogene produces a component of the cell membrane receptor for the epidermal growth factor [6]. Ras proteins are essential for the induction of DNA synthesis. They act in the late G1-phase of the cell cycle. Thus, many of the oncogene products are factors which are involved in the regulation of cell growth and cell differentiation. It is plausible that an autonomous production of such factors by the activated oncogenes is of basic importance for the unrestrained proliferation of the tumour cells.

Oncogenes in genito-urinary tumours were first discovered in bladder cancer when cellular oncogenes of the ras family were identified in cell lines from patients with carcinoma of the bladder [7]. Expression of altered ras genes has also been identified in carcinoma of the prostate [8]. Ras proteins are believed to act by elevating the levels of intracellular cyclic adenosine monophosphate. It has been found that prostatic epithelial cells are regulated by cyclic adenosine monophosphate in cell culture [8]. It would then be justified to assume that elevation of cyclic adenosine monophosphate would promote cell proliferation *in vivo* as well.

Using an immuno-histochemical assay, Viola and co-workers [9] identified a ras oncogene protein in prostate cancer cells. This protein was found only occasionally in low grade cancer but in all high grade lesions. They found this protein to be more reliable in tumour detection than carcino-embryonic antigen or prostate-specific antigen, and the only marker of the 3 that reflected the grade of malignancy.

It is known that prostate cancer tissue contains less acid phosphatase than normal or hyperplastic prostate [10]. Li and coworkers [11] found that prostatic acid phosphatase is a phosphotyrosine protein phosphatase. It may then be assumed that the reduction of acid phosphatase activity in the malignant prostate may lead to enhanced concentration of phosphotyrosine proteins with a consequent stimulation of cell proliferation.

In addition to ras genes, a number of other proto-oncogenes have been identified in prostate cancer. Rijnders and co-workers [12], who studied cell lines from 4 human prostate cancer tumours grown in nude mice, found expression of a myc gene in large amounts in all 4 cell lines. Cellular myc, like fos, belong to a set of oncogenes whose products are localized in the nucleus and involved in the cell cycle. These genes have the ability to immortalize cells in cell culture, that is, to provide them with the capacity to replicate indefinitely. When cultured cells are used for studies on carcinogenesis, the cells must be immortalized to transform to malignant behaviour. It may be presumed that a related kind of action may have importance for malignant transformation *in vivo*. Rijnders et al. also found that the expression of different proto-oncogenes reacted in different ways on the presence or absence of testosterone in the medium. It is known that oncogenes may interact with hormones like estrogen and testosterone.

Our present knowledge of the oncogenes and their function can probably be summarized in the following way:

The cell growth and cell replication are regulated by a number of growth factors, some of which have been identified. Their action is mediated by specific receptors on the cell surface. Under physiologic conditions the stimulation and inhibition of the growth process is regulated by the need of tissue regeneration. There is a balance between stimulation and inhibition.

The production of growth factor may lose its normal control and become unrestrained with the consequence that supernormal amounts of the factor are exported from the cell. If the cell carries receptors for this particular growth factor on its surface, an autonomous growth process, i.e., an autocrine process, may be the result.

Another possible factor may be a defect in the receptor. Normally the receptor mediates signals into the cell only on stimulation from an external growth factor. There can probably occur a defect in the receptor itself, resulting in a continuous sending of signals into the cell.

A third alternative is believed to be abnormal intracellular formation of growth stimulating products or abnormal reaction on hormones.

The process of cell growth is dependent on a system of growth factors and receptors, which influence each other. In the light of modern tumour biology, the development of cancer is evoked not by a sudden and solitary change of a cell or cells, but by a net-work condition where different cell systems are involved, and a step-wise procedure, maybe a step-wise activation of different cellular oncogenes.

It is well known that prostate cancer may express a highly variable progressive potential from being a very slowly growing, so-called latent cancer, to a rapidly growing cancer with a tendency to early dissemination. Some authors have recently postulated [13,14] that there is in fact only one variety of prostate cancer which has a slow growth rate with a logarithmic growth curve and with dissemination occurring usually only after a certain tumour volume has developed. They believe the biological malignant potential increases with increasing size of the tumour and that this increasing aggressiveness is also reflected in the cytomorphological appearance of the tumour. These statements are based on observations on rather small series of patients and the hypothesis still remains unproven.

Tumour Markers and Monoclonal Antibodies

Tumour markers

With the aim of identifying tumour markers for prostate cancer, much effort has been made to produce monoclonal or polyclonal antibodies against prostate-associated antigens. Tumour markers in serum can be of value to
i) detect disease,
ii) follow progression or regression of the disease, and
iii) serve as a prognostic marker. In human prostatic cancer a serum marker might be superior to a tissue marker, because of the marked heterogeneity of prostate cancer. Substances secreted into the circulation may better reflect the activity of the entire tumour.

Recent advances in protein purification and the elaboration of mono- and polyclonal antibodies have focused research interest on a number of cell antigens. Immuno-assay techniques have simplified clinical studies and made them rapid and safe.

Prostatic acid phosphatase (PAP) has been used for over 50 years as a marker in prostatic cancer [15]. Its main use has been in monitoring disease progression and regression following various forms of treatment. With the old enzymatic technique a raised value was almost invariably an indication of generalized disease. With the new immuno-assay techniques elevated levels of PAP may also be found in localized cancer [16,17]. The hope that PAP might be used as a general screening test for prostate cancer has not yet become reality [18]. On the other hand, PAP has proven to be a marker for tumour aggression: patients with elevated levels at the time of diagnosis had a worse prognosis than those with normal levels [19,20]. PAP is not organ-specific though. We have recently shown that PAP is secreted from the kidneys and, what is more, in equal amounts in males and females [21].

More recently, new markers have been identified. Prostatic antigen (PA) or prostate-specific antigen (PSA), as it is more often called, is a well defined glucoprotein and distinct from PAP [21,22]. PSA can not be used for screening of prostatic carcinoma but is reported to be superior to PAP in detecting early relapse of disease [23]. Also its prognostic reliability appears superior. In a series of over 1,000 patients with localized disease, PSA was given a p-value of 0.0002 using Cox's regression model, compared with 0.0684 for PAP [24]. In data from our own group based on approximately 100 patients and using bivariate analysis, PSA had a p-value of 0.0063, compared with 0.0014 for PAP [25] (compare Figs. 1 A and B). Siddall and coworkers [26], in a series of 91 prostate cancer patients found PSA as well as gamma-seminoprotein, another antigen of prostatic origin, superior to PAP in monitoring progression of the disease.

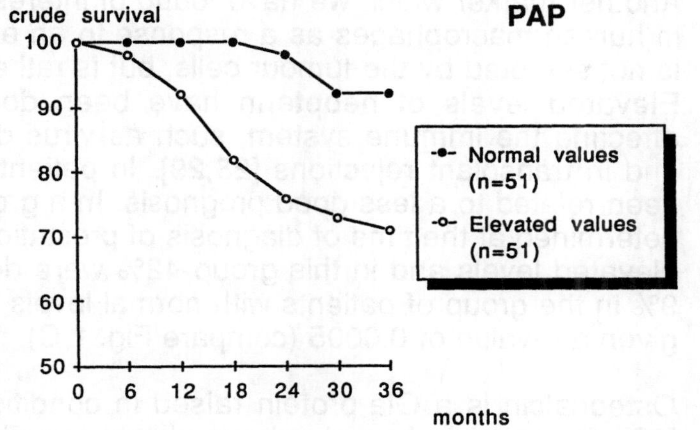

Fig. 1A

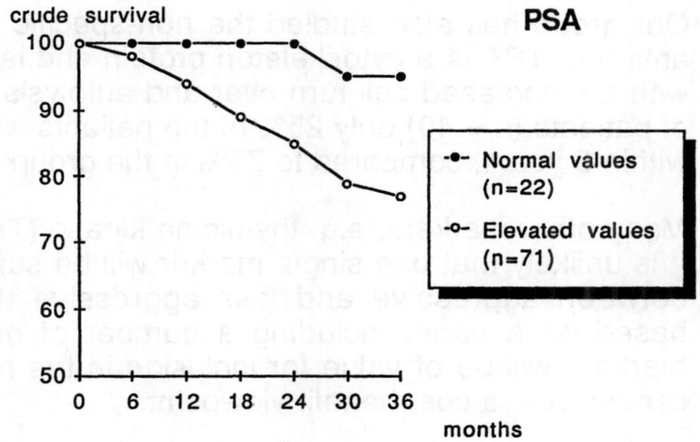

Fig. 1B

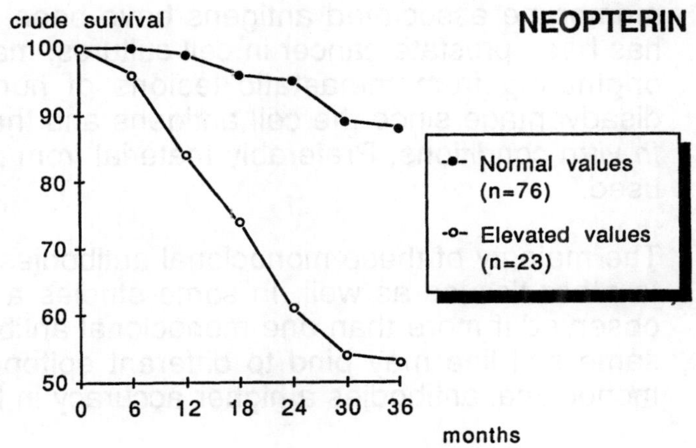

Fig. 1C

Another marker which we have found of interest is neopterin. Neopterin is synthesized in human macrophages as a response to an evoked immuno-response [27]. Hence, it is not secreted by the tumour cells, but is rather a host reaction to antigen production. Elevated levels of neopterin have been demonstrated in a number of diseases affecting the immune system, such as virus diseases, AIDS, autoimmune disorders, and in transplant rejections [28,29]. In patients with malignancies raised levels have been related to a less good prognosis. In a group of 93 patients neopterin levels were determined at the time of diagnosis of prostatic carcinoma. Twenty-seven per cent had elevated levels and in this group 42% were dead within 3 years, compared with only 9% in the group of patients with normal levels [30]. In bivariate analysis neopterin was given a p-value of 0.0005 (compare Fig. 1 C).

Osteocalcin is a Gla-protein raised in conditions with increased osteoblastic activity [32]. Osteocalcin has also been shown to reflect tumour activity. In our series 2-year survival for patients with elevated levels was only 43% as compared to 92% for the patients with normal serum content of osteocalcin [32]. In the same study referred to above [26], osteocalcin was ascribed a p-value of 0.0007 in bivariate analysis.

Our group has also studied the non-specific tumour marker TPA (tissue polypeptide antigen). TPA is a cytoskeleton protein and is excreted in large amounts in conditions with an increased cell turn-over and autolysis [33,34]. We found that in a small group of patients (n = 40) only 25% of the patients with normal values were dead from cancer within 5 years, compared to 75% in the group with elevated levels [20].

Many other markers, e.g. thymidine kinase (TK), are currently under investigation [35]. It is unlikely that one single marker will be sufficient to act as a safe guide in deciding between aggressive and less aggressive therapy. The decision will probably be based on a panel including a number of markers. Future research will tell which markers will be of value for inclusion in the routine work-up of patients with prostatic cancer from a cost-benefit viewpoint.

Antibodies Against Cell Membrane Antigens

Using lymphocyte-hybridoma techniques a number of antibodies against cell membrane associated antigens have been produced. The origin of these antibodies has been prostate cancer in cell cultures, mainly the cell lines PC-3 and DU 145, both originating from metastatic lesions of human prostatic cancer. This is a certain disadvantage since the cell antigens and their stability may have been altered by the *in vitro* conditions. Preferably material from primary human prostate cancer should be used.

The majority of these monoclonal antibodies are not specific to prostate cells but bind to other tissues as well. In some studies a more potent binding to cancer cells was observed if more than one monoclonal antibody was used. Different antibodies to the same cell line may bind to different epitopes on the cell surface, giving a panel of monoclonal antibodies a higher accuracy in the identification of cancer tissue.

Immunolocalization

Antibodies towards secretory proteins of prostatic origin are also used for immunohistochemical examination. The main importance of this technique is to support the prostatic origin of metastatic disease. In this sense prostate-specific antigen has appeared to be more sensitive than prostatic acid phosphatase [36]. No relation has been found between the intensity of staining and tumour aggressiveness [37].

Specific Immunotoxin Therapy

It has been suggested that monoclonal antibodies could be useful in the treatment of cancer, either by using tumour-cell specific antibodies alone or combining the antibody with a cytotoxic agent. The principle of targeting toxic agents selectively to tumour tissue has been called the "magic bullet", a concept coined by Paul Ehrlich at the beginning of the century [38].

A number of monoclonal antibodies against prostate cancer cells have been produced but so far there have been very few attempts to use the antibodies for therapeutic purposes. Deguchi and co-workers [39] conjugated methotrexate to a monoclonal antibody specific for human prostatic acid phosphatase. The antibody-cytotoxin complex was found to have an antitumour effect *in vitro*. However, it was found that, following injection to mice, the immunotoxin complex accumulated not only in the prostate but in other organs as well, such as the liver, spleen and kidney. Acid phosphatase is secreted by the prostate cells and is not stable in those cells or on their cell membranes. A prerequisite for a satisfactory effect of immunotoxic therapy is that the target antigen has a stable binding to the cell surface.

Webb and co-workers [40] produced monoclonal antibodies by immunizing mice with cells from prostate carcinoma cell lines. By using radio-immunoassays, the monoclonal antibodies alpha Pro 13 and alpha Pro15 were found to bind specifically to prostate cancer cells and not to cells from other kinds of cancer or normal tissues. These antibodies could therefore be potential carriers of cytotoxic substances. A ricin A-chain was used as toxin.

When the toxin was bound to the antibody by means of a chemical technique, a certain destruction of the monoclonal antibody occurred with a reduction of its binding capacity. A cell fusion technique was used to produce a specific immunotoxin consisting of a monoclonal antibody directed both against prostate cancer cells and against ricin A-chains. The ricin A-toxin was linked to the antibody by an antigen-antibody interaction, a hybrid immunotoxic conjugate.

The influence of the immunotoxin complex on the viability of prostate cancer cells was studied by calculating the inhibition of 14-C amino-acid uptake in the cultured cells. It was found that exposure to the immunotoxin complex produced a marked reduction of the 14-C amino-acid uptake in the cancer cells, whereas exposure to the monoclonal antibody alone or to the ricin A-toxin had no such inhibiting effect.

It was also found that, if the hybrid immunotoxic conjugate was added to the cell culture in combination with a chemotherapeutic agent like bleomycin, there was a

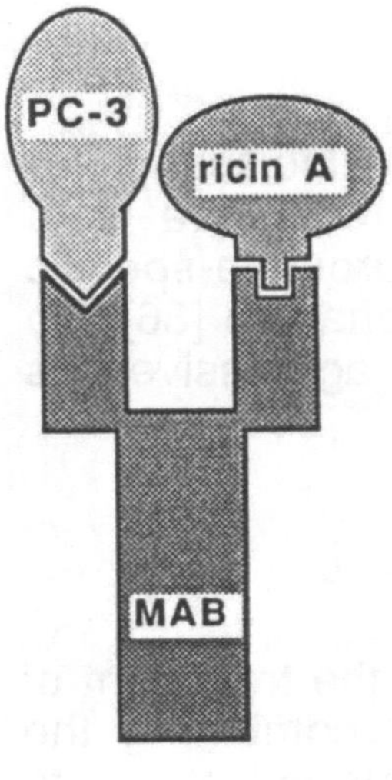

Fig. 2. Immunotoxin complex. The monoclonal antibody (MAB) directed against both the prostate cancer cell line PC-3 and ricin A-chain carries the toxin to the tumour cells.

synergistic effect: the 14-C aminoacid uptake was further reduced. The same synergistic effect was observed with methotrexate and vinblastine.

Hence, there is some evidence that immunotoxin therapy may be effective *in vitro*. However, a number of obstacles to the clinical use of the principle still remain. Most of the antibodies against prostate cancer cells bind to normal and hyperplastic prostate tissue as well and many of them even to other tissues. In addition, when the antibody-toxin conjugate has exerted its cell-killing effect, hopefully in the tumour tissue, there remains the risk of escape of the toxin moiety with subsequent cell-killing effect in other tissues.

Therefore, even if the preliminary results of this research appear promising, further investigation is necessary before we can be convinced that the "magic bullet" is a clinical reality.

REFERENCES

1 Anderson JR: Tumours:II. The aetiology of cancer. In: Muir's Textbook of Pathology. Edward Arnold, London. 1985, p 13.1

2 Horan Hand P, Thor A, Wunderlich D, Muraro R, Caruso A and Schlom J: Monoclonal antibodies of predefined specificity detect ras gene expression in human mammary and colon carcinomas. Proc Natl Acad Sci 1984 (81):5227

3 Hunter T and Sefton BM: The transforming gene product of Rous sarcoma virus phosphorylates tyrosine. Proc Natl Acad Sci 1980 (77):1311

4 Kirschenbaum A and Droller MJ: Update on oncogenes and relevance in urology. Urology 1987 (29):121

5 Doolittle RF: Simian sarcoma virus oncogene, v-sis, is derived from the gene (or genes) encoding a platelet-derived growth factor. Science 1983 (221):275

6 Downward J: Close similarity of epidermal growth factor receptor and V-erb - B oncogene protein sequences. Nature 1984 (307):521

7 Pacadas LF, Tabin CJ, Shih C and Weinberg RA: Human EJ bladder carcinoma oncogene is homologue of Harvey sarcoma virus ras gene. Nature 1982 (297):474

8 Peehl DM and Stamey TA: Oncogenes; a review with relevance to cancers of the urogenital tract. J Urol 1986 (135):897

9 Viola MV, Fronowitz F, Oravez S, Deb S, Finkel G, Lundy J, Hand P, Thor A and Schlom J: Expression of ras Oncogene p 21 in prostate cancer.N Engl J Med 1986 (314):133

10 Woodard QH: Quantitative studies of beta-glycerophosphatase activity in normal and neoplastic tissues. Cancer 1956 (9):352

11 Li HC, Chernoff J and Kirschenbaum MA: A phosphotyrosinylprotein phosphatase activity associated with acid phosphatase from human prostate gland. Eur J Biochem 1984 (138):45

12 Rijnders AWM, van der Korput JAGM, van Steenbrugge GJ, Romijn JC and Trapman J: Expression of cellular oncogenes in human prostatic carcinoma cell lines. Biochem Biophys Res Commun 1985 (132):548

13 Mc Neal JE, Bostwick DG, Kindrachuk RA, Redwine EA, Freiha FS and Stamey TA: Patterns of progression in prostate cancer. Lancet 1986 (I):60

14 Isaacs JT: Pre-malignant changes in the prostate - an animal model. Prostate 1985 (7):228

15 Gutman EB, Sproul EE, Gutman AB: Significance of increased phosphatase activity at the site of osteoplastic metastases secondary to carcinoma of the prostate gland. Am J Cancer 1936 (28):485

16 Vihko P, Lukkarinen O, Kontturi M, Vihko R: Effectiveness of radio-immunoassay of human prostate-specific acid phosphatase in the diagnosis and follow-up of therapy in prostatic carcinoma. Cancer Res 1981 (41):1180

17 Lewenhaupt A, Ekman P, Eneroth P, Eriksson A and Nordström L: Serum levels of prostatic acid phosphatase (PAP), tissue polypeptide antigen (TPA), CA-50, neopterin, and of osteocalcin in patients with prostatic carcinoma. Scand J Clin Lab Invest 1985 (45 Suppl 179):75

18 Gittes RF: Serum acid phosphatase and screening for carcinoma of the prostate. Editorial retrospective. N Engl J Med 1983 (309):852

19 Scardino PT, Seale C, Carlton EC: The prognostic significance of enzymatic prostatic acid phosphatase in clinically localized prostatic cancer. J Urol 1984 (131, part 2) Abstract 220, p 158A

20 Lewenhaupt A, Ekman P, Eneroth P, Nilsson B and Nordström L: Tissue polypeptide antigen (TPA) as a prognostic aid in human prostatic carcinoma. The Prostate 1985 (6):185

21 Nordström L, Ekman P, Eneroth P and Lewenhaupt A: Isoenzyme pattern of prostatic acid phosphatase in serum, urine, and homogenates from men and women. Scand J Clin Lab Invest 1985 (45 Suppl 179):89

22 Wang MC, Loor RM, Li SL and Chu TM: Physico-chemical characterization of prostate antigen purified from human prostate gland and seminal plasma. IRCS Med Sci 1983 (11):327

23 Killian CS, Lang N, Emrich LJ, Vargas FP, Kuriyama M, Wang MC, Slack NH, Papsidero LD, Murphy GP and Chu TM: Prognostic importance of Prostate Specific Antigen for monitoring patients with stages B2 to D1 prostate cancer. Cancer Res 1985 (45):886

24 Killian CS, Emrich LJ, Vargas FP, Yang N, Wang MC, Priore RL, Murphy GP and Chu TM: Relative reliability of five serially measured markers for prognosis of progression in prostate cancer. JNCI 1986 (76):179

25 Lewenhaupt A, Ekman P, Eneroth P and Nilsson B: Reliability of PAP, PSA, TPA, Neopterin, Osteocalcin, CA-50, TK, CRN, tumour grade and stage in predicting prognosis in human prostate cancer (submitted)

26 Siddall JK, Shetty SD and Cooper EH: Measurements of serum gamma-seminoprotein and prostate specific antigen evaluated for monitoring carcinoma of the prostate. Clin Chem 1986 (32):2040

27 Huber C, Fuchs D, Hausen A, Margreiter R, Reibnegger G, Spielberger M and Wachter H: Pteridines as a new marker to detect human T cells activated by allogenic or modified self major histocompatibility complex (MHC) determinants. J Immun 1983 (130):1047

28 Margreiter R, Fuchs D, Hausen A, Huber C, Reibnegger G, Spielberger M and Wachter H: Neopterin as a new biochemical marker for early diagnosis of renal allograft rejection: experience based upon evaluation of 100 consecutive cases. Transplantation 1983 (36):650

29 Goebel FD, Erfle V, Piechowiak H, Hien P, Schloz H and Hehlman R: The relations of HTLV-III antibodies to neopterin and beta-2-microglobulin in the serum of patients with AIDS or persons at risk. In:Biochemical and Clinical Aspects of Pteridines, Vol 4. De Gruyter, Berlin 1985 p 319

30 Lewenhaupt A, Ekman P, Eneroth P, Eriksson A and Nordström L: Neopterin as a prognostic aid in prostatic carcinoma. Eur J Urol 1986 (12):422

31 Deftos J, Parthermore G & Price A: Changes in plasma bone Gla-protein during treatment of bone disease. Calif Tissue Int 34:121, 1982.

32 Lewenhaupt A, Ekman P, Eneroth P, Kallner A and Nordström L: Tumour Markers in Human Prostatic Carcinoma. On optimation of reference values. (in press).

33 Lüning B and Nilsson U: Sequence homology between TPA and intermediate filament proteins. Acta Chem Scand 1983 (37 B):731

34 Skryten A, Unsgaard B, Björklund B and Englund G: Serum TPA related to activity in a wide spectrum of cancer conditions. Tumor Diagn 1981 (3):117

35 Gronowitz JS, Källander CFR, Diderholm H, Hagberg H and Pettersson V: Application of an in vitro assay for serum Thymidine Kinase: Results on viral disease and malignancies in humans. Int J Cancer 1984 (33):5

36 Stein BS, Petersen RO, Vangore S and Kendall AR: Immunoperoxidase localization of prostate specific antigen. Am J Surg Pathol 1985 (6):553

37 Lewenhaupt A, Collins P and Ekman P: Immunohistochemical localisation of prostatic acid phosphatase, prostate specific antigen, and of tissue polypeptide antigen in human prostatic carcinoma (submitted)

38 Ehrlich P: Collected Studies on Immunity. John Wiley, New York 1906

39 Deguchi T, Chu TM, Leong S, Horoszewicz JS and Lee C: Effect of methotrexate-monoclonal anti-prostatic acid phosphatase antibody conjugate on human prostate tumour. Cancer Res 1986 (46):3751

40 Webb K, Ware J and Paulson DF: A review: prostate monoclonal antibodies - the magic bullet. Urology 1986 (4):193

The Endocrinological Basis for Hormonal Therapy

M. Motta

Department of Endocrinology, University of Milan, Italy

The basis of all endocrine investigations related to the prostate is provided by the observation that the growth and the activity of the normal gland is largely dependent upon androgens, a characteristic which is frequently retained by the prostatic cells undergoing development into neoplastic cells (70% of all cases of prostatic tumors). This concept is supported by the fact that castrated patients very seldom develop tumors of the prostate.

Since the fundamental observation of Huggins and his colleagues [1,2], establishing the hormone dependence of prostatic cancers, the treatment of these diseases is essentially aimed either at inhibiting androgen secretion or at interfering with their action at the prostatic level. Endocrine therapy of carcinoma of the prostate includes orchidectomy, hypophysectomy, adrenalectomy, administration of estrogens, of progestagens, treatment with androgen antagonists (antiandrogens or inhibitors of androgen biosynthesis and metabolism) and, more recently, administration of potent, long-acting agonistic analogs of LHRH, either alone or in combination with antiandrogens .

A better understanding of the mechanisms through which each of the several endocrine treatments exhibits its antitestosterone effects, is of fundamental importance for the optimal clinical utilization of the drugs.

This chapter will first summarize the roles played by the different hormones involved in the regulation of the function of the prostate. Then the mode of action, through which the different endocrine treatments are based, will be presented. Attention will be paid not only to the therapeutical approaches which have already been tested with promising results in clinical trials, but also to the more recent ones, which are expected to be of clinical significance. It is not the aim of this chapter to discuss the choice of the most effective, safe and least troublesome method from the various endocrine regimens available, or to indicate which patients would benefit from endocrine treatments. These 2 points will be dealt with in other chapters of this volume.

Endocrine Regulation and Physiology of the Prostate

Androgens

Androgens play a central role in the complex process of the control of prostatic function and growth (see Figs. 1 and 3). The primary source of androgens are the testes, but a small contribution comes also from the adrenals. The testes secrete about

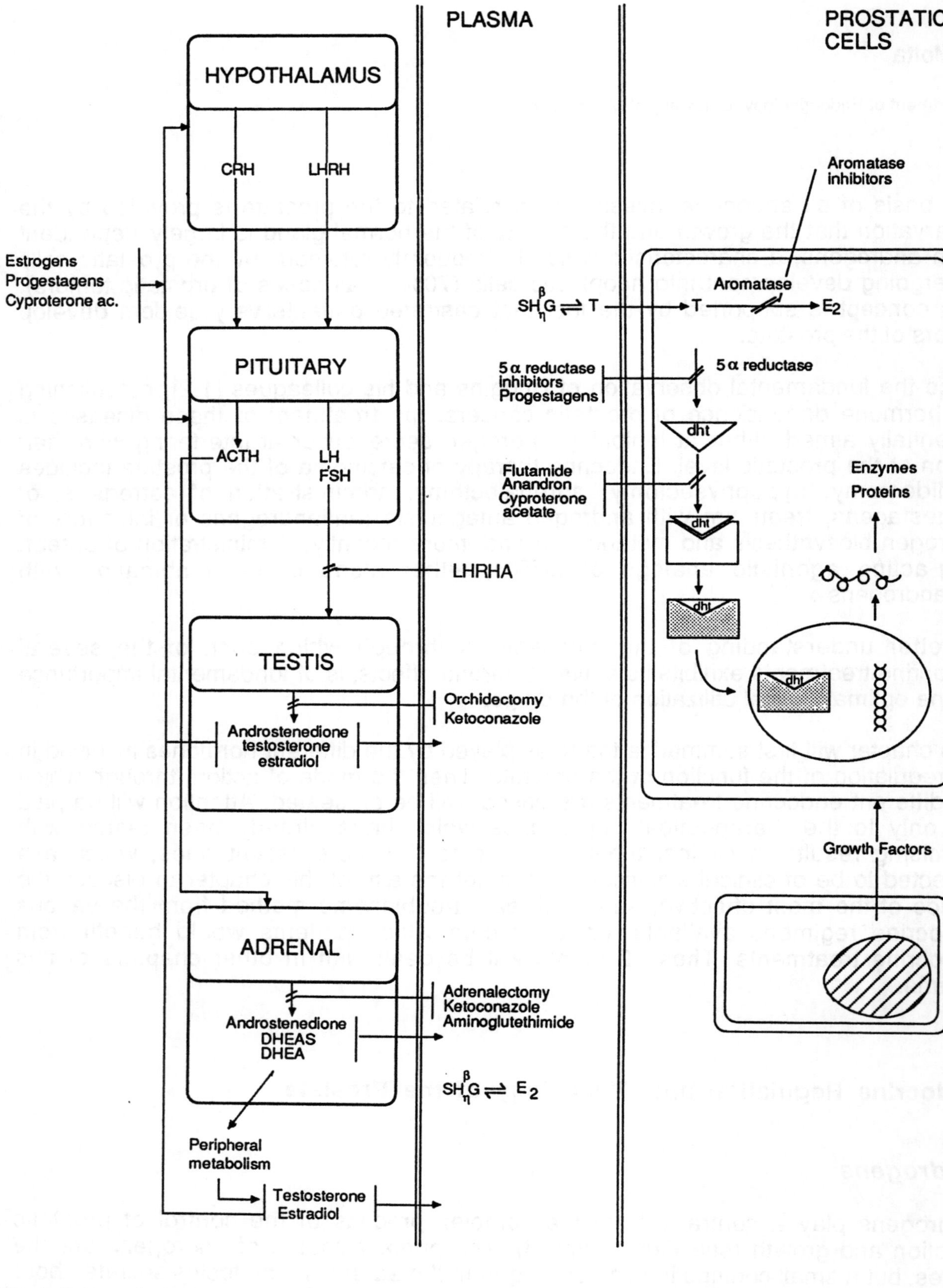

Fig. 1. Schematic representation of the endocrine control of the function of the prostate

5 to 10 mg of testosterone per day and also contribute approximately 30% of the plasma androstenedione either by a direct secretion or, indirectly, by peripheral conversion of testosterone [3]. In plasma, testosterone is reversibly bound to the steroid hormone binding globulin (SHBG), so that only about 2% of total plasma testosterone remains in a free unbound state; it is this free fraction which is considered to be the biologically active form of the hormone [3].

Androgens of testicular origin (in particular testosterone) are synthesized and released by the Leydig cells in response to stimulation by luteinizing hormone (LH). This pituitary hormone is, in turn, controlled by the hypothalamic LH releasing hormone (LHRH), which is secreted into the hypophysial portal circulation and reaches the anterior pituitary. To promote the release of the gonadotropins (LH and follicle stimulating hormone or FSH), LHRH binds to specific receptors localized on the membrane of the gonadotropic cells. Plasma levels of testosterone in turn regulate the release of both LHRH and gonadotropins by a negative feedback mechanism, thought to operate both at the hypothalamic and the pituitary level [4].

The main androgens of adrenal origin (which account for about 10% of the total amount of circulating androgens) are dehydroepiandrosterone (DHEA), its sulphate (DHEAS) and androstenedione. These steroids undergo metabolic conversion to testosterone and dihydrotestosterone (DHT), either in plasma or in the prostate itself (see below); data are available which indicate that the human prostatic tissue appears to have the ability to take up and metabolize adrenal androgens [5]. The adrenal production of androgens is controlled by adrenocorticotropic hormone (ACTH), which is under the influence of the hypothalamic corticotropin releasing hormone (CRH).

Recently, adrenal androgens have been assigned a role in promoting tumor growth [6,7]. The concept that the adrenals may influence prostatic growth and function received support from the work of Tullner [8], who found that the administration of ACTH to immature castrated rats promoted the growth of the ventral prostate, while there was no response in adrenalectomized animals. However, a recent study of the group of Walsh [9] indicates that, in patients with hypogonadotropic hypogonadism, but with normal adrenal glands, the prostates at autopsy are very small and atrophic. These contradictory findings suggest that it is still a matter of debate whether adrenal androgens are as important as those of testicular origin in favoring the growth of prostatic tumors.

<u>Metabolism and mechanism of action of androgens</u>. At prostatic level testosterone does not act as such, but needs to be converted into different 5-alpha-reduced metabolites. A large group of *in vitro* and *in vivo* studies has unequivocally established that the prostate, as other androgen-sensitive peripheral structures (seminal vesicles, sebaceous glands, etc.), metabolizes testosterone into 5-alpha-androstane-17-beta-ol-3-one (DHT), 5-alpha-androstane-3-alpha, 17-beta-diol (3-alpha-diol), and 5-alpha-androstane-3-beta, 17-beta-diol (3-beta-diol) [10-12]. These conversions occur under the influence of an enzymatic complex which includes a 5-alpha-reductase and 2 alpha- and beta-hydroxysteroid dehydrogenases. In the prostate, testosterone is also converted to delta-4-androstenedione, 5-alpha-androstanedione and androsterone (see Fig. 2). These metabolic processes have been extensively studied in animal models. It is likely that testosterone is metabolized in a similar manner by the normal prostatic tissue; however, the difficulty of obtaining normal human material for these types of studies is self-evident.

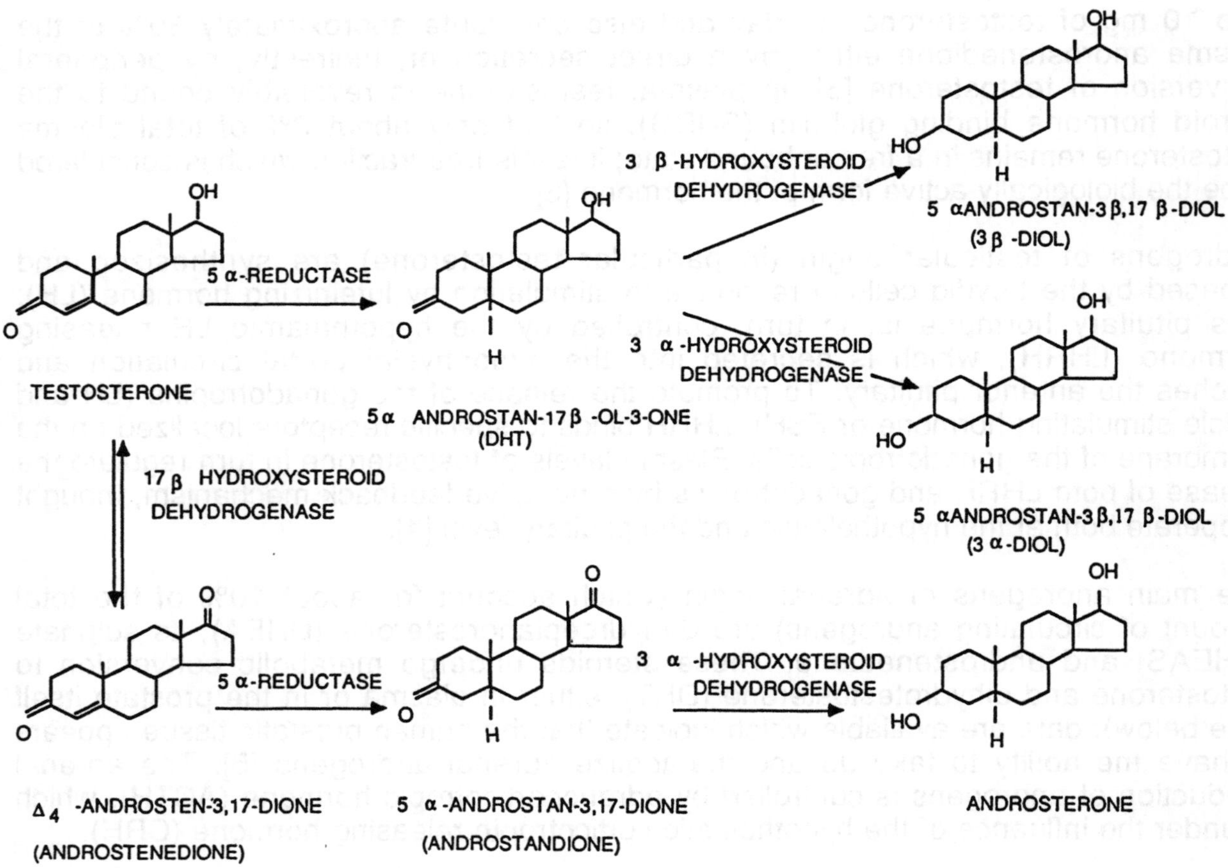

Fig. 2. Schematic representation of the metabolism of testosterone

Studies on the mechanism of action of androgens in the prostate demonstrate the important role of the conversion of testosterone to DHT, and indicate this hormone as the active intracellular androgen upon which the growth and the function of the prostate depends [13,14]. To exert its influence on cell function, DHT has to be taken up and bound to a specific receptor in the cytosol. Cytosol receptors have been shown to be present in the normal prostate [15,16]. Subsequently, the receptor undergoes a process of activation which allows translocation of the steroid hormone to the nucleus of the cell. The receptor-hormone complex binds to an acceptor site located on the chromatin and directs the transcription of stored genetic material by increasing synthesis of specific messenger RNAs, which, in turn, lead to the specific response of the cell (growth, secretion, etc.).

DHT represents also the predominant steroid hormone in the diseased prostate; BPH is frequently associated with high tissue accumulation of DHT and increased tissue 5-alpha-reductase activity [17,18]. On the contrary, in malignant tissue the 5-alpha-reductase activity and the formation of DHT seem to be considerably diminished; in this disease, testosterone metabolism appears predominantly to follow the oxidative pathway with the formation of androstenedione [19] (see Fig. 2). Also androgen receptors are present in the pathological prostate and retain the characteristics of those present in normal cells [20].

Estrogens

Other steroid hormones, such as estrogens, also seem to be involved in the control of the function of the prostate. Estrogens, which originate from the aromatization of androgens, are produced in small amounts by testicular tissue, but may also derive from the peripheral conversion of androstenedione of adrenal and testicular origin. Similarly to testosterone, estradiol is bound to SHBG and, through a negative feedback mechanism, influences the release of both LHRH and gonadotropins [4] (see Fig. 1).

Although the exact role of estrogens in the prostate has not been fully established, they have been shown to stimulate, either by themselves or in synergism with androgens, prostate growth and secretion [21,22]. These observations, coupled with the finding that receptors for estrogens are present in the prostate [16, 20], seem to suggest that these hormones act directly upon the gland.

Increasing evidence indicates that estrogens may also participate in the development of BPH [18,23]; it has also been reported that the tissue concentration of estrogens is higher in the malignant gland than in BPH [24]. Support for the possible involvement of estrogens in the pathogenesis of prostatic diseases comes from the recent study of Stone and his colleagues [25] who have found that the prostate has the capability to aromatize androgens to estrogens. Whether the *in situ* formation of estrogens is more relevant than the estrogens derived peripherally from the precursors in BPH, still remains to be established.

Peptide Hormones

Peptide hormones are also capable of influencing the growth of the prostate. Those most studied are prolactin and growth hormone (GH); more recently, the tissue growth factors have also received some attention.

<u>Prolactin.</u> The secretion of prolactin is mainly regulated by an inhibitory influence from the hypothalamus; the prolactin inhibiting factor is presently identified with dopamine. Once this is released into the hypophysial portal vessels, it inhibits the secretion of prolactin [26]. On the other hand, estrogens and TRH (thyrotropin releasing hormone) stimulate prolactin secretion; estrogens appear to act via central nervous regulatory centers [26] (see Fig. 3). Hyperprolactinemia is frequently observed in prostatic cancer patients under estrogen treatment [27].

Prolactin exerts its effects
1) on the testes, where it acts synergistically with LH to stimulate testosterone secretion [28];
2) on the adrenals, where it promotes the release of DHEA, DHEAS and androstenedione [29], and
3) via a recently suggested [30] direct mitogenic action on prostatic cells, where receptors for this pituitary hormone have been localized [31]. As a consequence of this, prolactin may promote the growth of the prostate independently of androgen action. Prolactin may also enhance the responses of the prostate to androgens, by acting synergistically with testosterone in promoting the growth of the gland, and influence the uptake of testosterone and the intraprostatic metabolism of androgens

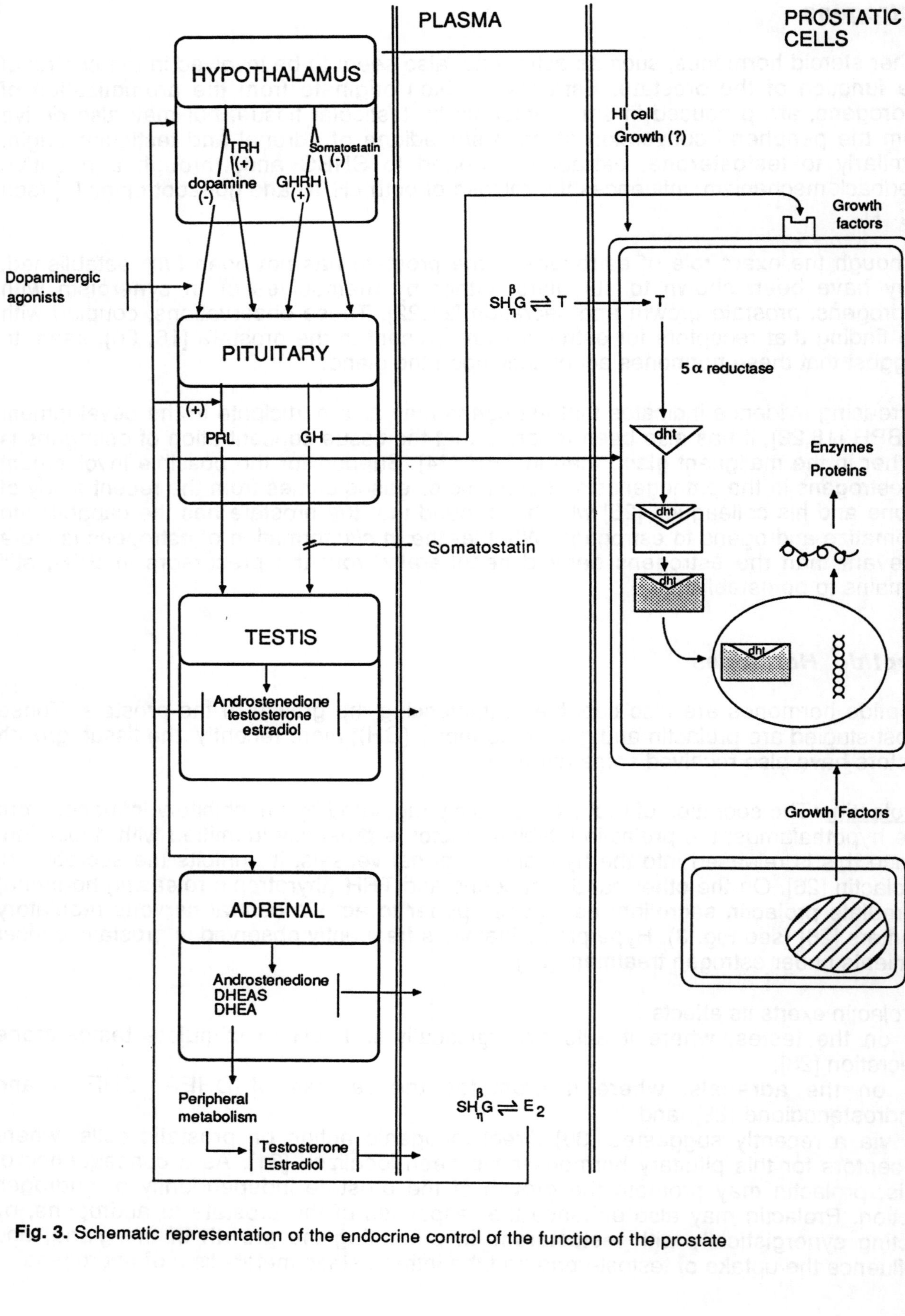

Fig. 3. Schematic representation of the endocrine control of the function of the prostate

[31,32]. On the basis of these observations, it is presently believed that prolactin plays a regulatory role in the growth, maintenance and function of the prostate.

Prolactin also seems to exert similar effects on the pathological human prostate. A higher and faster uptake of testosterone has been observed to occur in BPH patients whose plasma prolactin levels have been stimulated with chlorpromazine, when compared with untreated subjects [33]. However, because of the complexity of its actions, the involvement of prolactin in the development and maintenance of prostatic cancer is far from being completely understood.

GH. The secretion of GH is regulated by 2 hypothalamic hormones, one stimulating (GHRH, Growth Hormone Releasing Hormone) and one inhibiting (GHIH, Growth Hormone Release Inhibiting Hormone, somatostatin) (see Fig. 3). The growth promoting action of GH is mediated by the somatomedins, a group of structurally related polypeptides (see below), which seem to exert a negative feedback effect on GH release by stimulating somatostatin secretion, and by a direct effect on the pituitary where they block the action of GHRH [34]. Since GH appears to be the major regulator of plasma somatomedin levels, it might be expected that the effects of GH on the prostate are mediated by the somatomedins.

The possible participation of GH in the control of prostatic growth is still insufficiently understood. However, the observations that the administration of GH and ACTH to hypophysectomized castrated rats stimulates prostatic growth [35] and that GH levels are higher in patients with metastatic prostatic cancer than in patients without metastases [36], indicate that this hormone plays a role in the progression of the tumor. This is supported by recent findings showing that GH is localized in human prostatic tumors [37] and that this tissue possesses specific binding sites for GH [37].

Tissue growth factors. Tissue growth factors, which include many peptides (epidermal growth factor, EGF; transforming growth factor, TGF; nerve growth factor, NGF; somatomedins, etc.), form a class of regulatory molecules possessing potent mitogenic activity. They exert their effects by binding to specific receptors present on the cell surface and by acting through a paracrine mode of action. Additionally, since these factors have biological effects on the same cell where they are produced and their receptors are present, they are able to stimulate cellular growth in an autocrine fashion [38]. The importance of growth factors and of their receptors in cancer is stressed by the finding that 3 oncogenes are in fact the genes coding for one growth factor and 2 receptors.

The purification and partial characterization of a prostate-derived growth factor secreted by prostatic tissue with the potential to mediate some of the activities related to prostatic growth and development, suggests selective roles of mitogenic growth factors in prostatic neoplasia [39].

In addition, a potent mitogen for prostate epithelial growth (Prostatropin) has been isolated from bovine brain [40] and is supposed to have a role in the function of the prostate. It has still to be understood how these factors fit in amongst the other systems of hormonal control of prostatic growth and how they are involved in the malignant transformation of cells. Further studies on how these substances interact will probably provide further insight for the development of new types of treatment of prostatic tumors.

Mechanism of Action of the Different Therapeutic Approaches

The endocrine control of the growth and function of the normal prostate is a complex process, the crucial event of which is to maintain an adequate supply of androgens, in particular testosterone, to the gland. It is not yet totally clear how many of the factors involved in such a regulation (see above) are also equally responsible for the growth and evolution of prostatic tumors. At any rate, the dependence upon testosterone of many of the prostatic tumors is undoubted. Therefore the rationale of every endocrine treatment in prostatic cancer is either to lower testosterone levels in the general circulation or to interfere with the metabolism and the biological effects of the hormone at cellular level. As it will be shown below, the mode of action of each hormonal manipulation is quite different, since they operate at different levels of the endocrine regulation of prostatic function.

Bilateral Orchidectomy

The most conventional and direct method to maximally lower plasma androgen levels is to remove the primary source of testosterone by bilateral orchidectomy. After removal of the testes, it can be predicted that any residual testosterone in the circulation is of adrenal origin. Secondary endocrine effects occur after orchidectomy: as expected, these principally involve the hypothalamo-pituitary axis with a permanent increase of plasma levels of LH and FSH, as a consequence of the loss of the negative feedback effect exerted by testosterone on LHRH and gonadotropin secretion (see Fig. 1).

Estrogens

Drugs with estrogenic properties are thought to act principally by inhibiting the activity of the hypothalamo-pituitary system through a negative feedback mechanism (see Fig. 1). This effect leads to a fall in the secretion of LH, which results in the decrease of testosterone synthesis by testicular tissue [4].

It must be pointed out that estrogenic compounds may also, acting directly at the testicular level, decrease the synthesis of testosterone, and exert a direct local action on the prostate, as indicated by a decrease in the intraprostatic conversion of testosterone to DHT, by an inhibition of DNA synthesis etc. [41-43]. It must, however, be underlined that estrogenic drugs develop their antitumoral action mainly because of their feedback effect on the hypothalamo-pituitary axis. All the other effects occur when estrogens are given in doses far exceeding the levels that can be achieved in patients without any marked side effects.

As previously mentioned, estrogenic compounds increase plasma prolactin levels. This secondary effect could be relevant while treating patients with prostatic cancer, since prolactin is able to influence the growth of the prostate, as reported in the preceding section. However, on the basis of the available clinical studies, it is unlikely that the doses of estrogens used can induce an increase in plasma prolactin levels capable of affecting adrenal and/or testicular synthesis of androgens.

Estrogenic drugs utilized to treat prostatic cancers are either non-steroidal synthetic compounds (such as diethylstilbestrol, diethylstilbestrol diphosphate, chlorotrianisene and dienestrol) or steroids (such as polyestradiol phosphate or estradurin, and ethinylestradiol). It is obvious that the ideal agent of this type for the treatment of prostatic cancer should have predominantly an antigonadotropic activity and a local antiandrogenic effect on prostatic tissue, but minimal estrogenic side effects.

Progestagens

Progestational drugs, the most studied of which are megestrol acetate and medrogestone [18,44], exhibit their effects directly on the hypothalamo-pituitary axis (see Fig. 1); via a negative feedback mechanism they inhibit LH release, thereby decreasing testicular secretion of testosterone [18]. Similarly to progesterone, they also prevent the transformation of testosterone to DHT, possibly by acting as preferential substrates for the 5-alpha-reductase. A decrease in the intraprostatic concentrations of DHT, and a blockade of the 5-alpha-reductase activity are thus achieved [18,44-46]. Unlike estrogens, progestagens do not increase serum levels of prolactin.

Androgen Antagonists

A more modern method of depriving prostatic cancer tissue of its trophic stimulus, testosterone, is based on the utilization of androgen antagonists. This class of substances includes both the antiandrogens and the inhibitors of androgen biosynthesis and metabolism.

Antiandrogens. Antiandrogens (such as cyproterone acetate, flutamide, anandron, etc.) are compounds that block the biological effects of testosterone within the target organ cell, by inhibiting the binding of DHT to its receptors [47]. The antiandrogen-receptor complex does not translocate into the cell nucleus, and consequently the hormonal effect on protein synthesis is prevented (see Fig. 1). Because of their mechanism of action, the antiandrogens are able to counteract the effect of androgens of both testicular and adrenal origin.

Despite the fact that antiandrogens have basically the same mechanism of action, their *in vivo* endocrine effects are quite different. A distinction is generally made between those substances which also have other endocrine properties (e.g. progestational and antigonadotropic activities) and the pure antiandrogens which have only antiandrogenic properties.

To the first category of antiandrogens belongs cyproterone acetate. Since this compound possesses a strong progestational effect, it induces a reduction of plasma LH and FSH levels, by activating the negative feedback mechanism at the hypothalamo-pituitary level, and consequently it inhibits the biosynthesis of testicular androgens [48]. At the same time, this steroid competes with androgens for the same receptors at the target cell [48]. Thus, androgen deprivation in the case of cyproterone acetate is obtained in 2 ways: 1) by inhibition of androgen biosynthesis through the suppression of gonadotropin secretion, and 2) by inhibition of the remaining (adrenal) androgens by an action at the receptorial level (see Fig. 1).

In contrast to cyproterone acetate, pure antiandrogens, such as flutamide and anandron, are devoid of progestational and antigonadotropic properties [49,50]. They only compete with androgens at their receptor sites at the level not only of the prostate, but also of the hypothalamo-pituitary complex (where androgens exert their negative feedback effect) (see Fig. 1); as a result, LH secretion is increased and consequently, in the presence of the testes, the biosynthesis of testosterone is also increased [51]. However, the hormone, because of the presence of the antiandrogen, cannot exert its action in the prostate.

Since these 2 classes of antiandrogens express their effects *in vivo* in a different way, this implies that they also have different clinical applications. Only antiandrogens of the cyproterone acetate type should be suitable for the so-called monotherapy in non-castrated patients, while both types of antiandrogens should be useful when given in combination with castration. Cyproterone acetate seems to be more appropriate than pure antiandrogens in the initial phase of treatment with LHRH agonists, because it inhibits, at least partially, the oversecretion of testosterone (see below). Both types of antiandrogens should be equally qualified in combination with LHRH therapy after "down regulation" of the pituitary LHRH receptors has occurred (see below).

Inhibitors of androgen metabolism. So far the approach of antagonizing the effects of androgens has been only that of displacing androgens from their specific receptor sites. The demonstration that DHT and estrogens are the mediators of trophic effects in the prostate and that 5-alpha-reductase and aromatase are the enzymes involved in the intracellular transformation of testosterone into DHT and estrogens respectively (see above), may provide the basis for the development of new androgen antagonists. It is obvious that in the presence of these compounds testosterone reaches its target structure but is unable to exert its activity because of the absence of the intracellular transformation into DHT and estrogens. 5-alpha-reductase inhibitors and aromatase inhibitors belong to this new class of androgen antagonists.

5-Alpha-reductase inhibitors. Progesterone, megestrol acetate, medrogesterone have all been reported to inhibit 5-alpha-reductase [18,44,45]. However, these compounds possess other endocrine properties which prevail over that of inhibiting 5-alpha-reductase activity. Compounds whose primary mode of action is that of interfering with this enzyme have now been tested both *in vivo* and *in vitro* in different animal tissues [12,13,52,53]. It has been reported that, when given *in vivo*, they selectively inhibit testosterone, but not DHT-induced growth of the prostate of castrated rats [13] as well as of dogs [54]. However, these molecules have not been tested yet in clinical trials, because of the lack of adequate pharmacological and toxicological studies. When more detailed studies have been performed, the selective inhibitors of 5-alpha-reductase may certainly represent another opportunity for the treatment of prostatic diseases.

Aromatase inhibitors. Aromatase inhibitors are those compounds which block the transformation of androgens to estrogens interfering with the aromatase activity [55]. Since estrogens have been suggested as playing a role in the development of prostatic cancers [18,23-25], it is conceivable that these compounds may prove useful in the treatment of these diseases. Particular attention has been paid to one of these molecules, namely 4-hydroxy-androstenedione; preliminary studies indicate that this compound is effective in prostatic diseases [55].

The approach of interfering with the metabolism of testosterone either with the 5-alpha-reductase inhibitors or with the aromatase inhibitors presents definite advantages over the other types of treatment, because they suppress the effect of testosterone at the target level, but leave the plasma concentrations of the hormone unmodified. Of course much work has to be done yet, but the results are very promising.

LHRH Analogs

A radically different and novel endocrine approach for depressing androgenic stimulation of prostatic cancer is represented by the use of highly potent long-acting LHRH analogs. These compounds became available soon after the structure of LHRH has been elucidated [56]. Two different categories of LHRH analogs have been synthesized: 1) the superactive agonists which possess marked biological and pharmacological activities with a more prolonged duration of action, but in which the full pattern of activity of the original hormone is maintained; and 2) the antagonistic analogs which are devoid of any intrinsic LHRH activity, but which are able to inhibit the activity of endogenous LHRH by interacting with its receptors at the pituitary level.

<u>LHRH agonists.</u> The most potent agonistic analogs of LHRH show the substitution of the amino acid in position 6 with a D amino acid (biodegradation is thus prevented), and the deletion of the amino acid in position 10 with the addition of an ethylamide group to the proline residue in position 9 (a higher affinity to receptors is thus achieved) [57].

The peculiarity of these analogs is that, depending on the doses and on the modality of administration, they are able both to stimulate and to inhibit gonadotropin secretion. Acute and pulsatile administration of these analogs stimulates the secretion of gonadotropins and results in increased testosterone production by the testes. On the contrary, continuous administration of high doses of LHRH agonists causes an inhibition of LH and FSH release, and a subsequent suppression of testosterone secretion similar to that obtained by surgical castration [58] (see Fig. 4). The so-called "paradoxical" effect (antigonadic) exhibited by LHRH agonists has centered attention on the utilization of these compounds as antitumoral agents and has been proved valid both in animal and human studies [59].

The ability of chronic administration of LHRH agonists to totally suppress gonadotropin secretion occurs via the so called "down regulation" of the receptors for LHRH present at the pituitary level. As a result, the pituitary gland becomes refractory to further stimulation by LHRH analogs and testicular androgen production is then prevented [60]. However, it must be underlined that all LHRH agonists, irrespective of their molecular structure or of the way of administration (s.c., i.m., intranasal etc.), induce an initial and immediate hypersecretion of gonadotropins which is accompanied by an increase in testosterone release [58]. Only when plasma levels of the LHRH agonists are sufficiently elevated do the pituitary receptors become blocked, with down regulation and inhibition of gonadal function.

The pituitary gland does not seem to be the only target tissue for LHRH; extrapituitary effects have also been postulated. These include

1) an action on the testes where LHRH agonists interfere with the biosynthesis of testosterone, and down regulate LHRH receptors [58]. So far, however, this phenomenon has been demonstrated in several animal species, but not in humans [58];
2) a direct action on the prostate itself. Specific binding sites for LHRH seem to be present in prostatic tumors [61]. Despite the multiple sites of action, the pituitary gland is, however, believed to be the main target for LHRH agonists.

The therapy of prostatic cancer with LHRH agonists has 2 drawbacks: one is related to the initial stimulatory period, during which there is an exacerbation of the disease-related symptoms due to the hypersecretion of testosterone; the second is due to the fact that the LHRH therapy blocks testosterone coming from the testes, but is ineffective on androgens of adrenal origin. During therapy with LHRH agonists there are, therefore, persisting, although low, levels of androgens in the circulation [7]. One way to overcome these disadvantages is to give the LHRH therapy with an antiandrogen, which prevents the binding of endogenous testosterone to its own receptors at the prostatic level (see sections on antiandrogens and adrenal suppression).

LHRH antagonists. LHRH antagonistic analogs are mainly obtained either by removing the amino acid residue in position 2, or by substituting it with a D amino acid, and by introducing a D amino acid in position 6 [57]. Similarly to LHRH agonists, LHRH antagonists induce an inhibition of gonadotropin release and lower testosterone secretion, although their mechanism of action is totally different from that of the LHRH agonists [59]. These substances are biologically inactive and exert their effect at the receptor level by preventing the binding of the endogenous LHRH to its pituitary receptors. Preliminary evidence suggests that these compounds are able to

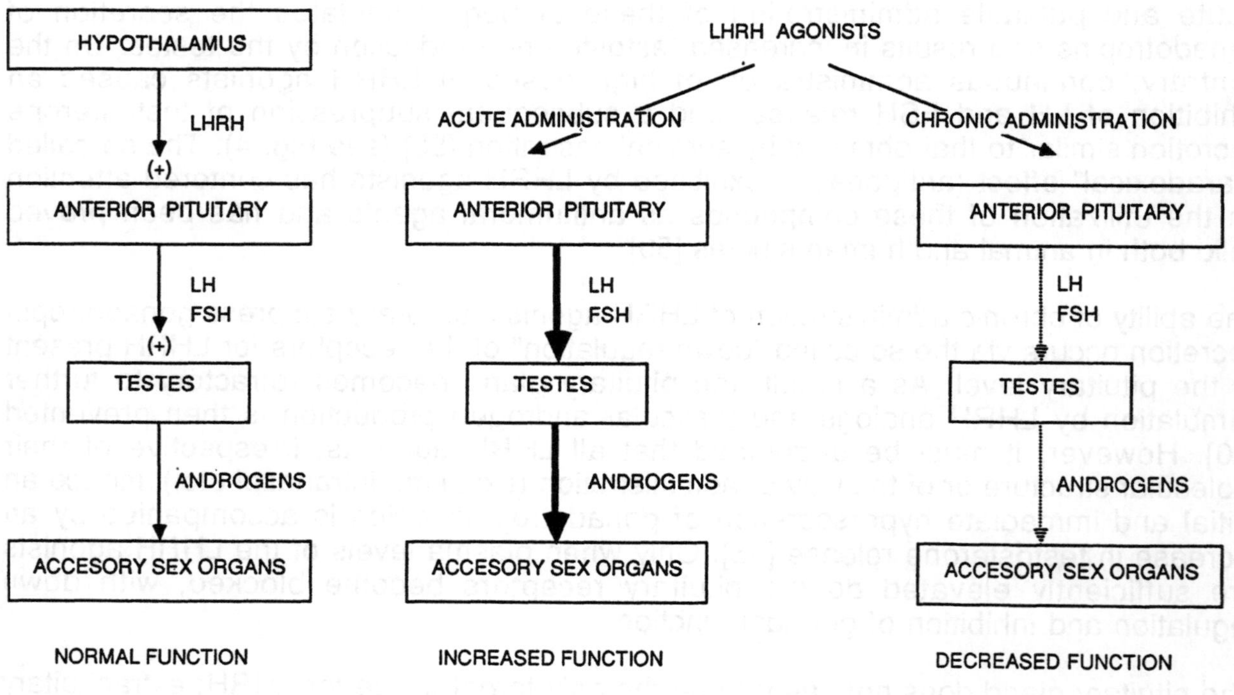

Fig. 4. Endocrine effect of acute and chronic administration of LHRH agonists

significantly reduce prostatic tumor size and growth [62]. Suppression of the Dunning prostate tumor growth has been obtained after chronic administration of LHRH antagonists [62]. In addition, the binding of one of the LHRH antagonists to plasma membrane obtained from the Dunning prostate tumor indicates that LHRH antagonists might also act directly on the prostate [61].

These preliminary experimental studies suggest that this class of compounds should also be considered for the therapy of prostatic carcinoma. Their use would avoid the transient stimulation of the release of gonadotropins and of testosterone which occurs initially in response to LHRH agonists, thus preventing the temporary flare-up of the disease [59]. However, LHRH antagonists have been tried in humans only in acute studies, and clinical data are not yet available on the effects of their chronic administration. As soon as a complete toxicological investigation is performed, the LHRH antagonists may then represent another therapeutic approach for the future.

Since both LHRH agonists and antagonists have to be given in a continuous fashion, the development of long-acting pharmaceutical depot formulations appears an essential step for their optimal clinical application.

Adrenal Suppression

Measurements of intraprostatic concentrations of DHT have revealed unexpectedly elevated amounts of DHT in some prostatic carcinomas after orchidectomy, administration of estrogens or of LHRH agonists, although these treatments cause a 90% decrease in serum testosterone levels [7,63]. This finding suggests that significant amounts of adrenal androgens may be converted to DHT within the tumor tissue after suppression of testicular androgenic production and that the high tissue levels of DHT remaining after surgical or medical castration seem to have a stimulatory effect on the evolution of prostatic cancers [7]. However, the lowest amount of androgens capable of stimulating prostatic tumor growth is not yet well defined [64]. Nevertheless, this possibility stresses the need to neutralize the action of androgens of adrenal origin and gives support to the concept of total androgen suppression in the treatment of prostatic cancers. Specific pharmacological treatments for removing adrenal androgens are available.

Aminoglutethimide. Aminoglutethimide produces a medical blockade of adreno-cortical function, by inhibiting the side chain cleavage of cholesterol and subsequent hydroxylation, an early step in steroidogenesis. Consequently, the synthesis of androgens, cortisol and aldosterone is interrupted [65] (see Fig. 1). The deficiency of cortisol and aldosterone in the general circulation leads to a hypersecretion of ACTH from the pituitary gland and justifies the substitution therapy with hydrocortisone concomitant with aminoglutethimide.

Ketoconazole. Ketoconazole is an orally administered synthetic imidazole derivative that is used widely in the treatment of fungal diseases. High doses of this drug block the synthesis of testosterone in the testes and adrenal glands of animals and men [66] (see Fig. 1). Clinical studies with ketoconazole in prostatic cancers are limited and toxicity at the dose levels required is defined incompletely.

Total androgen suppression. The availability of new drugs or combinations of agents capable of suppressing the effect of both testicular and adrenal androgens has made possible the achievement of the so-called total androgen ablation in the treatment of prostatic cancers. Total androgen suppression theoretically can be achieved by excluding all sources of androgen production or by blocking all androgen effects at the target cell level. The most promising form of androgen ablation as first-line therapy for prostatic cancers appears to be the combination of LHRH agonists with an antiandrogen [7] (see above).

Somatostatin

Somatostatin, a 14 amino-acid containing cyclic peptide, was first isolated from the hypothalamus and subsequently found in the pancreatic islets and in the gut [67]. This hormone possesses several differing actions: it inhibits hormone secretion (GH, insulin, glucagon and possibly prolactin), DNA synthesis and cell proliferation [67].

Somatostatin itself seems to be of limited value in the therapy of human disorders. The 2 major problems that limit its therapeutic effectiveness are its short half-life after systemic administration (due to its rapid inactivation by peptidases) and its marked diversity of action (i.e., its lack of selectivity for a given target cell or tissue). Structural analogs of somatostatin have been synthesized in an effort to circumvent these problems [67].

Because somatostatin analogs possess the same properties as the native hormone, they might prove useful in treating certain forms of cancer, since they might suppress the growth and/or the secretory activity of tumors [67]. Preliminary findings may suggest a possible application of these analogs in the management of prostatic cancer. Low doses of these compounds have been shown to suppress the growth of Dunning R 3327 prostatic cancer [68].

It is not yet known through which mechanisms somatostatin analogs may interfere with the growth of cancer cells. They might act by decreasing prolactin release, a hormone which is implicated in promoting prostatic cell growth [68]; by suppressing the secretion of GH involved in prostatic cell growth; or by inhibiting the mitogenic effects of tissue growth factors. For istance, it has been shown that somatostatin analogs suppress EGF-induced cell replication [68]. In addition, based on the fact that somatostatin analogs block the secretion of the somatomedins which mediate the action of GH, and that somatomedin-like peptides are present in prostatic cells and act as mitogenic autocrine factors, it is possible to speculate that somatostatin analogs might interfere with the local production and/or secretion of somatomedins. These possibilities are not necessarily mutually exclusive.

Further studies are needed to clarify the link between these factors and hormonal effects; such studies might show whether an approach based on the control of other hormonal signals will be therapeutically applicable, and perhaps advantageous as compared to the more classical methods already available for prostatic cancer therapy.

Acknowledgements

Supported by CNR grants, through the Special Target Projects "Preventive and Rehabilitative Medicine" (contract No. 86.01871.56) and "Oncology" (contract No. 86.00473.44) and by funds from MPI.

REFERENCES

1 Huggins C and Hodges CV: Studies on prostatic cancer. The effect of castration, of estrogen and of androgen injection on serum phosphatases in metastatic carcinoma of the prostate. Cancer Res 1941 (1):293-297
2 Huggins C, Stevens RE Jr and Hodges CV: Studies on prostatic cancer. II. The effects of castration on advanced carcinoma of the prostate gland. Arch Surg 1941 (43):209-223
3 Vermeulen A: The androgens. In: Grey CH and James VHT (eds) Hormones in Blood. Academic Press, London 1979 (3):355-416
4 Piva F, Motta M and Martini L: Regulation of hypothalamic and pituitary function: long, short, and ultrashort feedback loops. In: De Groot LJ (ed) Endocrinology. Grume and Stratton, New York 1979 (1):21-33
5 Harper ME, Pike A, Peeling WB and Griffiths K: Steroids of adrenal origin metabolised by human prostatic tissue in vivo and in vitro. J Endocr 1974 (60):117-125
6 Labrie F, Dupont A and Belanger A: Complete androgen blockade for the treatment of prostate cancer. In: De Vita VT, Hellman S and Rosenberg SA (eds). Important Advances in Oncology. Lippincott, Philadelphia1985 pp 193-217
7 Labrie F, Dupont A, Belanger A and St Arnaud R: Treatment of prostate cancer with gonadotropin-releasing hormone agonists. Endocr Rev 1986 (7): 67-74
8 Tullner WW: Hormonal factors in the adrenal-dependent growth of the rat ventral prostate. NCI Monograph 1963 (12): 211-223
9 Oesterling JE, Epstein JI and Walsh PC: The viability of adrenal androgens to stimulate the adult human prostate: an autopsy, evaluation of men with hypogonadotropic hypogonadism and panhypopituitarism. J Urol 1986 (136):1030-1034
10 Krieg M, Bartsh W, Janssen W and Voigt KD: A comparative study of binding metabolism and endogenous levels of androgens in normal hyperplastic and carcinomatous human prostate. J Steroid Biochem 1979 (11):615-624
11 Bruchovsky N and Wilson JD: The conversion of testosterone to 5-alpha-androstan-17beta-ol-3-one by rat prostate in vivo and in vitro. J Biol Chem 1968 (243):2012-2021
12 Motta M, Zoppi S, Brodie AM and Martini L: Effect of 1,4,6-androstantriene-3,17-dione (ATD),4-hydroxy-4-androstene-3,17-dione (4-OH-A) and 4-acetoxy-4-androstene-3,17-dione (4-Ac-A) on the 5-alpha-reduction of androgens in the rat prostate. J Steroid Biochem 1986 (25):593-599
13 Brooks JR, Baptista EM, Berman C, Ham EA, Hichens M, Johnston DBR, Primka RL, Rasmusson GH, Reynolds GF, Schmitt SM and Arth GE: Response of rat ventral prostate to a new and novel 5-alpha-reductase inhibitor. Endocrinology 1981 (109):830-836
14 Blohm TR, Laughlin ME and Benson HD: Pharmacological induction of 5-alpha-reductase deficiency in the rat: separation of testosterone-mediated and 5-alpha-dihydrotestosterone-mediated effects. Endocrinology 1986 (119):959-966
15 Fang S and Liao S: Androgen receptors. Steroid-and-tissue specific retention of 17-beta-hydroxy-5alpha-androstan-3-one-protein complex by the cell nuclei of ventral prostate. J Biol Chem 1971 (246):16-24
16 Barrack ER and Coffey DS: The specific binding of estrogens and androgens to the nuclear matrix of sex hormone responsive tissues. J Biol Chem 1980 (255):7265-7275
17 Isaacs JT, Brendler CB and Walsh PC: Changes in the metabolism of dihydrotestosterone in the hyperplastic human prostate. J Clin Endocrinol Metab 1983 (56):139-146
18 Geller J: Benign prostatic hypertrophy: current understanding of its pathogenesis. In: Labrie F and Proulx L (eds) Endocrinology. Excerpta Medica, Amsterdam 1984 pp 909-912
19 Smith CB, Masters JRW and Ghamadian R: Differential androgen metabolism in prostatic tumors. J Endocr 1980 (85):5-6
20 Kirdani RY, Emrich LJ, Pontes EJ, Priore RL and Murphy GP: A comparison of estrogen and androgen receptor levels in human prostatic tissue from patients with non-metastatic and metastatic carcinoma and benign prostatic hyperplasia. J Steroid Biochem 1985 (22):569-575
21 Thompson SA, Rowley DR and Heidger PM: Effects of estrogen upon the fine structure of epithelium and stroma in the rat ventral prostate gland. Invest Urol 1979 (17):83-89
22 Mawhinney MG and Neubauer BL: Actions of estrogen in the male. Invest Urol 1979 (16):409-420
23 Krieg M, Bartsch W, Thomsen M and Voigt KD: Androgens and estrogens: their interaction with stroma and epithelium of human benign hyperplasia and normal prostate. J Steroid Biochem 1983 (19):155-161
24 Ghanadian R and Puah CM: Relationship between oestradiol-17-beta, testosterone, dihydrotestosterone and 5-alpha-androstane-3-alpha, 17-beta-diol in human benign hypertrophy and carcinoma of the prostate. J Endocr

1981 (88):255-262
25 Stone NN, Fair WR and Fishman J: Estrogen formation in human prostatic tissue from patients with and without benign prostatic hyperplasia. Prostate 1986 (9):311-318
26 Thorner MO: Prolactin: clinical physiology and the significance and management of hyperprolactinemia. In: Martini L and Besser GM (eds) Clinical Neuroendocrinology. Academic Press, New York 1977(1):319-361
27 Jacobi GH and Wenderoth UK: New forms and future perspectives in endocrine treatment of prostatic carcinoma. Progress and Controversies in Oncological Urology. Springer Verlag, Berlin1980
28 Aragona C, Bohnet HG and Friesen HG: Localization of prolactin binding in prostate and testis: the role of serum prolactin concentration on the testicular LH receptor. Acta Endocrin 1977 (84):402-408
29 Jacobi GH: Palliativtherapie des Prostatakarzinoms. Endokrinologische Grundlagen, Klinische Situation, Prolaktinin neues Prinzip. Zuckschwerdt, München 1980
30 Smith C, Assimos D, Lee C and Grayhack JT: Metabolic action of prolactin on the prostate: independent of androgen action. Prostate 1985 (6):49
31 Boyns AR, Griffiths K, Pierrepoint CG and Peeling WB: Prolactin and the prostate. In: Goland M (ed) Normal and Abnormal Growth of the Prostate. Charles C Thomas, Springfield 1975 pp 431-444
32 Manandhar SF and Thomas JA: Effect of prolactin on the metabolism of androgen by the rat ventral prostate gland in vitro. Invest Urol 1976 (14):20-22
33 Farnsworth WE, Slannwhile WR, Jr and Sharma M: Interaction of prolactin and testosterone in the human prostate. Urol Res 1977 (15):83-91
34 Berelowitz M, Szabo M, Frohman LA, Firestone S and Chu L: Somatomedin-C mediates growth hormone negative feedback by effects on both the hypothalamus and the pituitary. Science 1981 (212):1279-1281
35 Lostroh AJ and Li CH: Stimulation of sex accessories of hypophysectomised male rat by non-gonadotrophin hormone of the pituitary gland. Acta Endocrin 1975 (25):1-16
36 British Prostate Study Group: Evaluation of plasma hormone concentrations in relation to clinical staging in patients with prostatic cancer. Brit J Urol 1979 (51):382-389
37 Sibley PEC, Harper ME, Peeling WB and Griffiths K: Growth hormonal and prostatic tumors: localization using a monoclonal human growth hormone antibody. J Endocr 1984 (103):311-315
38 James R and Bradshaw RA: Polypeptide growth factors. Ann Rev Biochem 1984 (53):259-292
39 Maehama S, Li D, Nauri H, Leykam JF and Denel TF: Purification and partial characterization of prostate-derived growth factor. Proc Natl Acad Sci USA 1986 (83):8162-8166
40 Crabb JW, Armes LG, Carr SA, Johnson CM, Roberts GD, Bordol RS and Mekeehan WL: Complete primary structure of prostatropin, a prostate epithelial cell growth factor. Biochemistry 1986 (25):4988-4993
41 Kirdani RY, Muntzing J, Varkarakis JM, Murphy GP and Sandberg AA: Studies on the antiprostatic action of estracyt, a nitrogen mustard of estradiol. Cancer Res 1974 (34):1031-1037
42 Hoisaeter PA: Incorporation of 3H-thymidine into rat ventral prostate in organ culture. Invest Urol 1975 (12):479-483
43 Daehlin L: On the effects of oestrogen in the male. Some effects of different oestrogenic substances in rats and men with prostatic carcinoma. Scand J Urol Nephrol 1985 (91, Suppl):21-35
44 Tan SY, Antonipillai I and Murphy BEP: Inhibition of testosterone metabolism in the human prostate. J Clin Endocrinol Metab 1984 (39):936-941
45 Massa R and Martini L: Interference with the 5-alpha-reductase system. Gynec Invest 1972 (2):253-270
46 Jagarinec N and Givner ML: Inhibition of testosterone metabolism of medrogestone in rat ventral prostate in vivo and in vitro. Archs Androl 1981 (7):39-44
47 Martini L and Motta M (eds): Androgens and Antiandrogens. Raven Press, New York 1977
48 Neumann F: Pharmacology and clinical uses of cyproterone acetate. In: Furr BJA and Wakeling AE (eds) Pharmacology and Clinical Uses of Inhibitors of Hormone Secretion and Action. Bailliere Tindall, London 1987 pp132-159
49 Neri R and Kassen N: Pharmacology and clinical uses of flutamide. In: Furr BJA and Wakeling AE (eds) Pharmacology and Clinical Uses of Inhibitors of Hormone Secretion and Action. Bailliere Tindal, London1987 pp160-169
50 Raynaud JP, Bonne C, Moguilewsky M, Levebvre FA, Belanger A and Labrie F: The pure antiandrogen RH 23908 (anandron), a candidate of choice for the combined antihormonal treatment of prostatic cancer: a review. Prostate 1984 (5):299-324
51 Neumann F, Habenicht UF and Schacher A: Antiandrogens and target cell response. Different in vivo effects of cyproterone acetate, flutamide and cyproterone. In: McKerns KW, Aakvaag A and Hansson V (eds) Regulation of Target Cell Responsiveness. Plenum Press, New York 1984 (2):489-527
52 Zoppi S, Cocconi M, Natali A, Costantini A, Serio M, Martini L and Motta M: In vitro effects of an aromatase inhibitor of 5-alpha-reductase activity in human hypertrophic prostatic tissue. J Clin Endocrinol Metab 1986 (63):269-271
53 Rasmusson GH: Biochemistry and pharmacology of 5-alpha-reductase inhibitors. In: Furr BJA and Wakeling AE (eds) Pharmacology and Clinical Uses of Inhibitors of Hormone Secretion and Action. Bailliere Tindall, London 1987 pp 308-325
54 Wenderoth UK, George FW and Wilson JD: The effect of a 5-alpha-reductase inhibitor on androgen-mediated growth of the dog prostate. Endocrinology 1983 (113):569-573
55 Habenicht UF, Scwartz K, Schweikert HU, Neumann F and El Etreby MF: Development of a model for the induction of estrogen-related prostatic hyperplasia in the dog and its response to the aromatase inhibitor 4-hydroxy-4-androstene-3,17-dione: preliminary results. Prostate 1986 (8):181-194

56 Baba Y, Matsuo M and Schally AV: Structure of the porcine LH-and FSH-releasing hormone. II. Confirmation of the proposed structure by conventional sequential analyses. Biochem Biophys Res Commun 1971 (44):459-461

57 Karten MJ and Rivier JE: Gonadotropin-releasing hormone analog design. Strucure-function studies toward the development of agonists and antagonists: rationale and perspective. Endocr Rev 1986 (7):44-66

58 Bhasin S and Swerdloff RS: Mechanisms of gonadotropin-releasing hormone agonist action in the human male. Endocr Rev 1986(7):106-114

59 Schally AV, Comaru-Schally AM and Redding TW: Antitumor effects of analogs of hypothalamic hormones in endocrine-dependent cancers. Proc Soc Exp Biol Med 1984 (175):259-281

60 Clayton RN and Catt KJ: Gonadotropin-releasing hormone receptors: characterization, physiological regulation and relationship to reproductive function. Endocr Rev 1981 (2):186-201

61 Hierowski MT, Altamirano P, Redding TW and Schally AV: The presence of LHRH-like receptors in Dunning R-3327H prostate tumors. FEBS Lett 1983 (154):92-96

62 Redding TW, Coy DH and Schally AV: Prostate carcinoma tumor size in rats decreases after administration of antagonists of luteinizing hormone-releasing hormone. Proc Natl Acad Sci USA 1982 (79):1273-1276

63 Geller J, Albert JD, Nachsheim DA and Loza D: Comparison of prostatic cancer tissue dihydrotestosterone levels at the time of relapse following orchiectomy or estrogen therapy. J Urol 1984 (132):693-696

64 Trachtenberg J: Optimal testosterone concentration for the treatment of prostatic cancer. J Urol 1985 (133):888-892

65 Worgul TJ, Santen RJ, Samojlik E, Veldhuis JD, Lipton A, Harvey HA, Drago JR and Rohner TJ: Clinical and biochemical effect of aminoglutethimide in the treatment of advanced prostatic carcinoma. J Urol 1983 (129):51-57

66 Sonino N: The endocrine effects of ketoconazole. J Endocrinol Invest 1986:341-347

67 Moreau JP and De Fendis FV: Pharmacological studies of somatostatin and somatostatin-analogues: therapeutic advances and perspectives. Life Sci 1987 (40):419-437

68 Defeudis FV and Moreau JP: Studies on somatostatin analogues might lead to new therapies for certain types of cancer. TIPS 1986(10): 384-386

Estrogens and Estramustine Phosphate

Lennart Andersson

Department of Urology, Karolinska Hospital, Stockholm, Sweden

In recent years estramustine phosphate (EMP) or Estracyt® has become an alternative to standard estrogen therapy in a number of centres. It has been debated whether estramustine is just one variant of estrogen or if it has another anticancer effect in addition.

This contribution provides a survey of what is known at present about the effects on prostate cancer of the various estrogenic drugs in clinical use, and of estramustine phosphate.

Prostate cancer is the tumour which is most responsive to hormone therapy. In 70-80% of the cases, progression of the disease is retarded for a longer or shorter period, if the testicular hormone production is eliminated. Following the fundamental discoveries by Charles Huggins in the 1930s and 40s that both the normal prostate and prostate cancer are androgen dependent [1], the principle of endocrine treatment for prostate cancer, usually with estrogens, was generally adopted and practised until the late 1960s and early 70s, when the Veterans Administration studies (VACURG) proved the hazards of estrogenic medication.

In the first VACURG study, 1903 patients with advanced prostate cancer, VA stages III and IV, were randomized to the following 4 groups:

Placebo
Diethylstilbestrol (DES) 5 mg/day
Orchidectomy + placebo
Orchidectomy + DES 5 mg/day.

Though the mortality from cancer was lower in the patients receiving DES, the death rate from cardiovascular disease was higher. Overall there were the same number of deaths in all groups [2].

In the second VACURG study, 508 patients with advanced prostate cancer were treated with DES at a dose of 0.2 mg/day, 1.0 mg and 5.0 mg/day or with placebo. In the patients given placebo or DES 0.2 mg/day there was a higher incidence of progression from stage III to IV than in the patients given 1.0 or 5.0 mg/day. In the groups on 1.0 and 5.0 mg/day there was a lower death rate from cancer than in the other groups, but the patients who received 5.0 mg had a higher rate of cardiovascular deaths. It could thus be concluded that DES in the dosage 0.2 mg/day was inadequate to control cancer, whilst DES 1.0 mg/day had a satisfactory anticancer effect without producing an excess of mortality from cardiovascular disease.

A number of investigations have shown that DES 3 mg/day is the minimum dose required to produce suppression of plasma testosterone to castrate level [3].

Increasing the dose of DES to 30 mg/day does not cause any further suppression of plasma testosterone. Regression of disseminated disease can thus be achieved even by submaximal testosterone depression. The dosage of DES most commonly used in clinical practice is 3 mg/day, although there has been a tendency in recent years to go down to a lower dosage, 1 or 2 mg/day.

The drugs with estrogenic properties which have been most commonly used in the treatment of prostate cancer include:

Diethylstilbestrol (DES), 1-3 mg /day p. o.
Diethylstilbestrol diphosphate (Honvan), 500 mg/day i.v. (10 days)
300-600 mg/day p.o.
Dienestrol, 5 mg/day p.o.
Chlorotrianisene (TACE), 12-24 mg/day p.o.
Ethinylestradiol, 150 microg/day p.o.
Polyestradiol phosphate, 40-80 mg/month i.m.

They have essentially the same inhibitory effect on the cancer. However, none of the other drugs has been so closely investigated with respect to the effect of various dosages as has DES.

Estramustine phosphate was constructed according to the so-called carrier principle. It is a combination of estradiol linked to nor-nitrogen mustard in the form of a carbamate. It was intended that, by binding to steroid hormone receptors, the drug should accumulate in the prostatic tissue and hopefully exert both a cytotoxic and hormonal effect. Pharmacokinetic studies in animals and in man have shown that EMP given orally is to a great extent dephosphorylated to estramustine in the gastrointestinal tract and further oxidized to estromustine [4, 5]. Part of the drug is metabolized to estradiol and estrone and the compound thus has an estrogenic action.

Following administration of estrogenic drugs or estramustine phosphate there is a significant and dose-dependent reduction of plasma testosterone, LH and FSH [6]. Thus EMP, like ordinary estrogens, has an antigonadotrophic effect.

The possible local effect of EMP in the prostatic tissue has been investigated in animal models and *in vitro*. The activity of 5-alpha-reductase in the prostate, causing the transformation of testosterone to 5-alpha-dihydrotestosterone, is significantly decreased, both in animals and in organ cultures of rat and human prostate tissue [7, 8]. It has also been shown that EMP inhibits the DNA-synthesis in the rat ventral prostate *in vitro* [9]. In cell culture, estramustine caused death of hormone unresponsive human prostatic carcinoma cells [10]. It has also been found to inhibit the growth of a number of animal tumours [11]. It has been shown by Hartley-Asp and others that the cytotoxic effect of EMP occurs by inhibition of microtubule function, the compound binding to microtubule-associated proteins with a disruption of the mitotic spindles and consequent mitotic arrest [12,13].

Estramustine and estromustine accumulate in the prostate, where they are bound to a cytosolic protein called estramustine-binding protein [14]. This protein has been detected in prostate cancer tissue with a tendency to higher levels in moderately well and poorly differentiated tumours than in well differentiated lesions [15]. No corresponding accumulation of the estrogenic moieties of EMP has been observed.

There is thus evidence that EMP, in addition to its estrogenic effect, has a direct action on the prostate cells and accumulates in the organ and the cancer tissue.

With regard to the possible local effects of estrogen on the prostate it has been shown that estradiol blocks the synthesis of testosterone from precursors and inhibits DNA polymerase *in vitro* [16]. It has also been shown that estradiol and ethinyl estradiol inhibit the release of testosterone from human testicular tissue *in vitro*, whereas this did not occur with DES [17]. All these effects occurred with the use of estrogen doses far exceeding the levels that can be achieved in man. There is no evidence of accumulation of estrogen in the prostate tissue. The drug Honvan (diethylstilbestrol diphosphate) was constructed with the aim that it should accumulate in the prostate but no such accumulation has been proven.

It must therefore be assumed that the effect of estrogens in the treatment of prostate cancer occurs primarily by a reduction of testicular androgen synthesis by inhibiting the pituitary gonadotrophin release - an androgen deprivation. Eriksson et al. [18] and others have shown that estrogen medication, like EMP, elevates the level of sex hormone-binding globulin in the plasma and also reduces the release of androgenic hormones of adrenal origin, dehydroepiandrosterone and dehydroepiandrosterone sulfate. This will probably cause a further reduction of the physiologically active free testosterone in plasma, a reduction which does not occur following orchidectomy.

EMP has been used as the primary treatment of prostate cancer in a number of open trials [19]. The clinical results in a number of such trials are summarized in Table 1.

As is seen in the Table, there was evidence of tumour remission in about 80% of the patients, which is similar to what is observed after standard estrogenic medication. In recent years the efficacy of EMP and the standard estrogen drugs in the primary treatment of prostate cancer has been compared in a number of controlled investigations (Table 2).

In 3 of the 5 investigations there was no significant difference between the 2 treatment modalities with respect to regression of the local tumour or metastatic deposits, relief of symptoms, or laboratory evidence of tumour remission. In the investigation of Benson and Gill [21] there was a longer time to progression in the patients on EMP therapy, and in a French multicenter study [23] EMP caused a superior relief of urinary tract obstruction and regression of metastatic lesions compared with DES. However, in neither of the trials was there any significant difference in survival between the 2 different protocols. On the other hand, there was a difference in the side effects.

Table 1. Effect of estramustine phosphate as primary therapy in prostate cancer in 17 phase II studies (from Edsmyr et al., 19)

Patients	Rate of tumour remission	
	Average	Range
340	82 %	60-100 %

Table 2. Controlled studies on EMP versus standard estrogen therapy in the primary treatment of prostate cancer

Authors	**Patients** No.	Categories	**Protocol**	**Results**
Andersson et al.[20]	182	T 2-4,M 0-1 G 1-2	EMP 840 mg/day Polyestradiol phosphate 80 mg/month + ethinyl estradiol 150 microg/day	No difference
Benson & Gill [21]	227	M 1,G 1-3	EMP 700-1,260 mg/day DES 3 mg/day	Longer time to progression in EMP group
Smith et al. [22]	227	T 3-4,M 0-1 G 1-3	EMP 560-->280 mg/day DES 3 mg/day	No difference
Hauchecome et al. [23]	115	T 2-3,M 0-1 G 1-3	EMP 420-1,120 mg/day DES 3-5 mg/day	Tumour regression superior in EMP group, especially in M 1 patients
Murphy et al. [24]	319	M 1, G 1-4	EMP 600 mg/m^2 daily DES 3 mg/day or orchidectomy cyclophosphamide + DES + 5 FU	No difference

It appears, therefore, that EMP and the so-called standard estrogenic drugs are of approximately equal value in the treatment of prostate cancer when the patient has been subjected to no prior hormonal manipulation or radiation therapy.

It is debatable whether EMP is superior to standard estrogens, or orchidectomy, in cases of poorly differentiated or anaplastic cancer. Leistenschneider and Nagel [25], in a series of 20 cases of poorly differentiated prostate cancer, observed cytomorphological evidence of tumour remission in 7 of 10 patients on EMP, but in only 1 of 10 on DES. On the other hand, in the studies by Benson and Gill [21] and by Smith et al. [22], EMP had no significantly superior effect in poorly differentiated cancer. The study by Andersson et al. [20] did not include G3 cases. The question whether EMP should be the drug of choice in poorly differentiated or anaplastic prostate cancer awaits further research. Some controlled investigations are going on.

EMP has been administered to patients with hormone refractory prostate cancer in a large number of studies (Table 3).

Table 3. Effect of estramustine phosphate in 34 phase II studies in patients with hormone refractory prostate cancer (from Edsmyr et al, 19)

Patients	**Rate of response to therapy** Average	Range
648	35 %	0-74 %

A response to the treatment was observed in 35% on average. The wide range of response rate may depend in part on differences in patient selection, but it probably also reflects the difficulties involved in the evaluation of progression and regression of deep tissue tumours where most of the lesions are not measurable or where the measuring techniques are inaccurate. However, a satisfactory effect was observed in about one-third of the cases.

Side effects following estramustine medication have been essentially the same and of the same frequency as with the standard estrogenic drugs. In some trials, cardiovascular complications occurred less frequently and were less severe with estramustine, particularly thromboembolic complications. On the other hand, nausea and vomiting occurred more often following EMP. In this context it should be stressed that many of the cardiovascular complications may be prevented or treated successfully by proper observation, with early prescription of diuretic drugs if signs of oedema occur, with anticoagulants for thromboembolic complications and with salicylic acid compounds or dipyridamole in threatening ischemic complications [26].

We would like to summarize our opinion on the use of standard estrogens and EMP in prostate cancer in the following way:

- In the absence of indications of tumour spread, hormonal manipulation or other kind of systemic treatment is rarely indicated. Therapy directed locally to the prostate should be preferred, such as surgery or irradiation, using an external or interstitial technique.

- In disseminated cancer there is reason to recommend androgen deprivation, at least if the patient has pain or other symptoms. We have the policy to start treatment in metastatic cancer even in the absence of symptoms, but we admit this is open to debate. We prefer orchidectomy to estrogen medication if it is acceptable to the patient, to avoid the risk of cardiovascular complications. However, low dose estrogen with close follow up with respect to untoward reactions is probably an equally good alternative. With respect to other modalities of androgen deprivation we refer to other sections of this book.

- In cases of poorly differentiated cancer estramustine may be superior to standard estrogenic drugs. However, a recommendation on this point should await further research.

- In prostate cancer which is, or has become, refractory to standard estrogens or orchidectomy, we consider estramustine phosphate the first therapeutic alternative, since there is probably a 35% chance that the patient will experience some relief and since the toxic effects are usually much less severe than after the ordinary cytotoxic drugs.

REFERENCES

1 Huggins C, Scott WW, Hodges CV: Studies on prostatic cancer. III The effects of fever, desoxycorticosterone, and of estrogen on clinical patients with metastatic carcinoma of the prostate. J Urol 1941 (46):997

2 Byar DP: The Veterans Administration Cooperative Urological Research Group's studies of cancer of the prostate. Cancer 1973 (32):1126

3 Scott WW, Menow M, Walsh PC: Hormonal therapy of prostatic cancer. Cancer 1980 (45):1929

4 Plym-Forshell G, Müntzing J, Ek A, Lindstedt E, Dencker H: The absorption, metabolism and excretion of Estracyt (NSC 89199) in patients with prostatic cancer. Invest Urol 1976 (14):128, 1976

5 Gunnarsson PO, Plym-Forshell G: Clinical pharmacokinetics of estramustine phosphate. Urology 1984 (23 Suppl 6):22

6 Jönsson G, Olsson A, Luttrop W, Cekan C, Purvis K, Diczfalusy E: Treatment of prostatic carcinoma with various types of estrogen derivatives. Vitamines and Hormones 1975 (33):351

7 Kadohama N, Kirdani RY, Murphy GP, Sandberg AA: 5-alpha-reductase as a target enzyme for anti-prostatic drugs in organ culture. Oncology 1977 (34):123

8 Kirdani RY, Müntzing J, Varkarakis JM, Murphy GP, Sandberg AA: Studies on the antiprostatic action of Estracyt, a nitrogen mustard of estradiol. Cancer Res 1974 (34):1031

9 Høisaeter PÅ: Incorporation of ^{3}H-thymidine into rat ventral prostate in organ culture. Invest Urol 1975 (12):479

10 Hartley-Asp B, Gunnarsson PO: Growth and cell survival following treatment with estramustine, nornitrogen mustard, estradiol and testosterone of a human prostatic cancer cell line (DU 145). J Urol 1982 (127):818

11 Müntzing J, Kirdani RY, Saroff J, Murphy GP, Sandberg AA: Inhibitory effects of Estracyt on R-3327 rat prostatic carcinoma. Urology 1977 (10):439

12 Hartley-Asp B: Estramustine induced mitotic arrest in two human prostatic carcinoma cell lines, DU 145 and PC-3. Prostate 1984 (5):93

13 Hartley-Asp B: Microtubule assembly in vitro as an aid in the study of aneuploidy. Aneuploidy I: Incidence and etiology. 1987 (in press)

14 Nelde HJ, Flüchter SH, Hartmann R, Bichler KH: Immunhistologischer Nachweis des Estramustin-bindenden Proteins (EMBP) in der Prostata. In: Harzmann et al (eds) Experimentelle Urologie. Springer Verlag. Berlin, Heidelberg 1985, p 332.

15 Flüchter SH, Nelde HJ, Björk P, Müntzing J, Bichler KJ: Estramustine-binding protein (EMBP) in human prostatic cancer tissue. Effect of anti-cancer treatment. 1987 (in press)

16 Harper ME, Fahmy AR, Pierrepoint CG, Griffiths K: The effect of some stilbestrol compounds on DNA polymerase from human prostatic tissues. Steroids 1970 (15):89

17 Daehlin L: On the effects of oestrogen in the male. Some effects of different oestrogenic substances in rats and men with prostatic carcinoma. Scand J Urol Nephrol. 1985 (Suppl 91):21

18 Eriksson A, Carlström K, Collste L: Estrogen treatment or orchidectomy in prostate cancer: Effects on testicular and adrenal androgens and on total androgen activity. (submitted)

19 Edsmyr F, Andersson L, Könyves I: Estramustine phosphate (Estracyt): Experimental studies and clinical experience. In: Jacobi and Hohenfellner (eds) Prostate cancer. Williams and Wilkins, Baltimore, London 1982, p 253.

20 Andersson L, Berlin T, Boman J et al: Estramustine versus conventional estrogenic hormones in the initial treatment of highly or moderately differentiated prostatic carcinoma. A randomized study. Scand J Urol Nephrol 1980 (Suppl 55):143

21 Benson RC, Gill GM: Estramustine phosphate compared with diethylstilbestrol. A randomized, double-blind, crossover trial for stage D prostate cancer. Am J Clin Oncol (CCT) 1986 (9):341

22 Smith PH, Suciu S, Robinson MRG et al: A comparison of the effect of diethylstilbestrol with low dose estramustine phosphate in the treatment of advanced prostatic cancer: Final analysis of a phase III trial of the European Organization for Research on Treatment of Cancer. J Urol 1986 (136):619

23 Hauchecorne J: Estramustine phosphate versus diethylstilbestrol. Etude comparative à propos de 115 malades. J Urol (Paris) 1987 (in press)

24 Murphy GP, Huben RP, Priore R: Results of another trial of chemotherapy with and without hormones in patients with newly diagnosed metastatic prostate cancer. Urology 1986 (28):36

25 Leistenschneider W, Nagel R: Estracyt therapy of advanced prostatic cancer with special reference to control of therapy with cytology and DNA-cytophotometry. Eur Urol 1980 (6):111

26 Hedlund PO, Gustafson H, Sjögren S: Cardiovascular complications to treatment of prostate cancer with estramustine phosphate (Estracyt) or conventional estrogen. A follow-up of 212 randomized patients. Scand J Urol Nephrol 1980 (Suppl 55):103

Antiandrogens

G.H. Jacobi

Urologische Klinik und Poliklinik, Johannes Gutenberg Universität, Mainz, Germany

A large number of both steroidal and non-steroidal compounds with antiandrogenic properties have been developed in the last 20 years. By far the most extensively investigated agent is cyproterone acetate, followed by flutamide and anandron. Only these 3 androgens play a clinical role in the palliative treatment of prostatic carcinoma today.

In urological circles the term 'andiandrogenic treatment' is often misused to include any type of contrasexual therapy such as estrogens, enzyme blockers or even LHRH analogues. However, andiandrogens in the strict sense of the word were defined by Dorfman [1] as: "substances which prevent androgens from expressing their activity at target sites". The inhibitory effect of these substances on androgen action must therefore be differentiated from compounds which inhibit the synthesis or release of pituitary hormones or which directly inhibit androgen synthesis in the gonads or the adrenals.

Mode of Action of Antiandrogens

The central mechanism of antiandrogenic action is competitive inhibition of the binding of dihydrotestosterone (DHT) to the cytosol receptor and, obviously, the inhibition of translocation of the activated DHT-receptor complex into the nucleus. The net effect is the reduction of nuclear concentration of DHT in androgen-dependent cells. As a consequence, androgen-dependent DNA synthesis is inhibited. Compounds which act exclusively in that way are called pure antiandrogens and include flutamide and anandron. They also inhibit the negative feedback effect of androgens at the hypothalamic centres, consequently increasing gonadotropin secretion and thus stimulating testosterone synthesis.

Cyproterone acetate, on the other hand, is not a pure antiandrogen since it possesses progestational, and thus antigonadotropic properties. This results in reduced gonadotropin stimulation with decreased biosynthesis of testicular androgen.

Biological Effects

Before antiandrogens were introduced in the treatment of patients with prostatic cancer, a number of sex-specific other effects were demonstrated in animal models. Antiandrogens cause atrophy and inhibition of secretory function of accessory sexual glands, such as the prostate and seminal vesicles, or involution of the epididymis and vas deferens. Spermatogenesis, libido and puberty are inhibited. In the androgen-supplemented castrated dog cyproterone acetate causes reduction in prostatic volume and secretion, as well as in RNA and DNA content of the prostatic cell [3].

The antitumoral effect of anandron has been proved in cell lines and in tumour models such as the hormone-sensitive rat Dunning tumour. The proof of efficacy of antiandrogens in the treatment of patients with prostatic carcinoma can only be given on clinical grounds, for 2 main reasons. Firstly, the androgen receptor content varies greatly from cancer to cancer and is usually unknown in the clinical situation. Secondly, the proof of the biological effect of andiandrogens *in vivo* as outlined above would require prostate biopsies and determination of nuclear DHT and nucleic acids. The advantage of the cyproterone acid-type antiandrogen is that, by its antigonadotropic action, the plasma testosterone is suppressed to about 1.5 ng/ml serum and can easily be monitored in patients under treatment. The advantage of the pure antiandrogen in maintaining serum testosterone and probably also sexual potency is commonly theoretical, at least in the majority of elderly patients in whom sexual function is either reduced or in whom sexual activity no longer plays any significant role.

Clinical Data

Cyproterone Acetate

Previous reviews of more than 300 patients treated with oral doses between 100 and 300 mg revealed that the interpretation of data was limited by several factors [4], including variations in treatment regimens, pretreatment evaluation, tumour staging and response criteria. In about half the cases cyproterone acetate was given as primary therapy in patients with newly diagnosed tumours, whereas in the others initial therapy (usually orchiectomy or estrogens) had failed before the antiandrogen was used. Overall, the striking clinical effect in previously untreated patients was regression of local tumour mass, improvement of the upper urinary tract, decrease of serum acid phosphatase, relief of bone pain, and improved performance.

Varenhorst [5] compared cyproterone acetate with orchiectomy and with estrogens in a randomised fashion. All 3 regimens were equally effective.

In a recent EORTC randomised trial Pavone-Macaluso et al. [6] have compared cyproterone acetate with medroxyprogesterone acetate and with the standard DES treatment. Local and distant tumour response, time to progression and survival did not differ significantly between patients treated with either the antiandrogen or the standard estrogen. However, cardiovascular side effects were less frequent with cyproterone acetate than with estrogen therapy.

When the intramuscular depot preparation became available, a randomised multicentre study was initiated in Europe. The intramuscular dose of 300 mg/week was compared with a standard estrogen regimen in a total of 191 patients [2]. Objective regression of local tumour after CPA was observed in 66%, an excellent to moderate histological regression being assessed upon rebiopsy in 57%. In terms of side effects CPA was superior to estrogens. Thus, cyproterone acetate can be considered as a valuable alternative to conventional estrogen treatment. Side effects are less, objective response rates are comparable and its value in certain estrogen-relapsed cases is documented.

Flutamide

In a review of antiandrogens in tumour therapy [2], patients treated with the non-steroidal pure antiandrogen flutamide were reviewed. Analysis of the data revealed the same pitfalls described in analysing the data on cyproterone acetate. An almost 50% response of varying degree was seen covering the same tumour sites and clinical parameters as mentioned before. In patients who were sexually potent at the time treatment was started, flutamide did not seem to hamper libido or potency.

More recently, Neri and Kassem [7] reviewed a randomised double-blind comparison between 1 mg per day DES and flutamide (750-1500 mg/day) for patients with previously untreated metastatic disease. A total of 125 patients were treated in 12 institutions for up to 102 weeks. By objective response criteria the efficacy of flutamide was equal to that of DES.

While gynaecomastia or breast tenderness and G.I. disturbances were equally distributed among the 2 groups, there was no cardiovascular complication in the flutamide group, as compared with 11.4% in the DES group.

Another randomised study compared the efficacy and side effects of flutamide (250 mg x 3) and estramustine phosphate (280 mg x 2) in 30 patients with metastatic cancer of the prostate. In a follow-up period ranging from 12 to 24 months, 13 out of 14 patients responded to flutamide and 11 of 12 patients on estramustine phosphate. However, 11 relapsed in the first group versus 2 in the second group, while 100% of the patients on estramustine phosphate lost their libido versus 20% of the patients treated with flutamide [8].

One last report deserves a mention in order to re-emphasize the difficulty of comparing data [9]. Seventy-two patients without previous hormone manipulation received 3x250 mg flutamide per day. The majority had had various palliative treatments of the local tumour or of metastases. Response criteria were not really comparable to those used by NPCP or the EORTC. On the basis of a never clearly defined overall 'favourable response' of 87.5%, the authors concluded that flutamide was a safe and usually effective drug for the treatment of advanced prostatic cancer.

From all the available and heterogeneous data it seems that there is no relevant clinical difference between the 2 antiandrogens so far described.

Anandron

The third antiandrogen covered in this chapter - anandron - is another non-steroidal compound clinically investigated more recently. Its mode of action is comparable to that of flutamide. Anandron has been used as an investigational drug predominantly in

France and Canada; other trials are being conducted at present in other European countries and in the USA. Anandron has never undergone any conclusive investigation as monotreatment, except in phase I toxicity studies. In doses between 50 and 900 ml/day, dose-related G.I. symptoms, anaemia or disturbance of light-dark adaptation may occur. The majority of the current anandron data derive from studies combining the drug either with orchiectomy or with LHRH analogues to achieve 'total androgen blockade'.

'Total Androgen Blockade' with the Use of Antiandrogens

This issue is covered in chapter 8. All 3 antiandrogens are used with the idea of 'neutralizing' the small amount of residual adrenal androgens left behind after surgical castration or LHRH agonist treatment. Unfortunately, this regimen has become prematurely elevated to an alternative 'standard treatment' in some European countries before early observations have been confirmed by randomised trials.

The Least Effective Dose of Antiandrogens

Since the inhibiting effects of antiandrogens at the androgen receptor site are competitive in nature, a severalfold preponderance of the antiandrogen is required to achieve a high inhibition of the intracellular androgen effect. For none of the aforementioned compounds has the least effective dose for clinical practice been established. In the light of toxicity as well as treatment costs this should be - among others - a challenge for the future.

Another challenge in the development of the non-steroidal antiandrogens is peripheral selectivity. The clinically utilised pure antiandrogens, flutamide and anandron, also inhibit androgen feedback at the hypothalamo-pituitary axis, thus effecting a stimulation of the testosterone secretion, which is undesirable. A new class of antiandrogens in preclinical development will act as a selective block in the accessory sex organs only [10].

REFERENCES

1 Dorfman RI: Biological activity of antiandrogens. Br J Dermatol 1970 (82 Suppl 6):3-8
2 Neumann F, Jacobi GH: Antiandrogens in tumor therapy. Clinics in Oncology 1982 (1):41-64
3 Tunn U, Senge Th, Schenck B, Neumann F: Effects of cyproterone acetate on experimentally induced canine prostate hyperplasia. A morhpological and histochemical study. Urol Intern 1980 (35):125-140
4 Jacobi GH, Altwein JE, Kurth KH, Basting R, Hohenfellner R: Treatment of advanced prostatic cancer with parental cyproterone acetate: a phase III randomised trial. Br J Urol 1980 (52):208-215
5 Varenhorst E: Metabolic changes during endocrine treatment in carcinoma of the prostate: a prospective study in man with special reference to cardiovascular complications during treatment with oestrogens, or cyproterone acetate or after orchiectomy. Linköping Univ Med Diss Nr 103
6 Pavone-Macaluso M, De Voogt H, Viggiano E, Barasolo E, Lardennois B, De Pauw M, Sylvester R: Comparison of diethylstilbestrol, cyproterone acetate and medoxyprogesterone acetate in the treatment of advanced

prostatic cancer: final analysis of a randomized phase III trial of the European Organisation for Research on Treatment of Cancer Urological Group. J Urol 1986 (136):624-631
7 Neri R, Kassem N: Pharmacological and clinical effects of antiandrogens. In: Agarwal MK (ed) Hormone Antagonists. De Gruyter, Berlin 1982
8 Johansson JE, Andersson SO, Beckham KW, Lingardh G, Zador G: Clinical evaluation of flutamide and estramustine as initial treatment of metastatic carcinoma of the prostate. Urology 1987 (29):55-59
9 Sogani PC, Vagaiwala MR, Whitmore Jr WF: Experience with flutamide in patients with advanced prostatic cancer without prior endocrine therapy. Cancer 1984 (54):744-750
10 Furr BJA: Novel antiandrogen: ICI 176, a pure peripherally selective, non-steroidal agent. J Endocrinol Invest 1987 (10 Suppl 2):13

Luteinizing Hormone Releasing Hormone Agonists

L. Denis

Department of Urology, A. Z. Middelheim, Antwerp, Belgium

The isolation and synthesis of the natural mammalian decapeptide luteinizing hormone-releasing hormone (LHRH) [1] was quickly followed by the synthesis of analogs, mainly by substitution of the sixth and tenth amino acids [2]. These analogs or agonists, sometimes surnamed superagonists, release more LH for longer periods of time due to the increased binding affinity to the LH receptors in the pituitary. The prolonged receptor occupancy by these agonists leads to desensitisation of the pituitary LH cell receptors with subsequent receptor loss, degradation of hormone receptor complexes and depletion of the LH pool. The observation that prolonged administration inhibited the growth of a prostatic tumor in a rat model and leads in men to inhibition of the gonadal steroid secretion initiated the interest in the utilisation of these drugs to treat human prostatic cancer [3]. This contribution reviews the recent advances obtained with these drugs in clinical experiments and practice.

Pharmacology of LHRH

Gonadotrophin secretion is physiologically regulated by intermittent pulses of LHRH. The biological effects of the agonists are identical to those induced by the natural LHRH, but their higher potency stimulates LHRH release for a few days in the initial phase followed by a decrease to base levels on continued chronic administration. This stimulation or acute release is dose dependent and adequate dosing or sustained release is necessary to obtain the inhibitory effect on the gonadal steroids [4].

The LHRH agonists have a wide range of clinical applications according to their stimulatory or suppressive activity, as presented in Table 1. The clinical application in

Table 1. Clinical indications for LHRH agonist therapy

Stimulatory activity:

- Hypogonadotrophic hypogonadism
- Idiopathic delayed puberty
- Cryptorchidism

Suppressive activity:

- Precocious puberty
- Endometriosis
- Breast cancer
- Contraception in females/males
- Prostate cancer

patients with prostatic cancer is mainly determined by its interference with the gonadotrophin release but extra pituitary activity has been reported in animal species by interaction with gonadal testosterone biosynthesis and the presence of LHRH receptors in rat prostatic tumors [5,6]. All agonists share the transient stimulation of gonadotrophin release which results in increased levels of serum testosterone in patients with normal gonads.

Antagonists, in contrast, reduce gonadotrophin secretions in humans immediately, thus preventing the initial elevation of the gonadotrophins caused by the agonists. Their clinical introduction is obstructed by the high doses necessary for treatment, the absence of the effect of desensitisation and high production costs [7].

The structures and trade names widely used in clinical experimentation and available for clinical practice are listed in Table 2. They all have the same N-terminal (Tyr) where the C sequence has been changed to nonapeptide ethylamide analogs or to decapeptide Aza Gly analog. They are classified in alphabetical order followed by their usual mode of administration by intranasal spray (IN), subcutaneous daily injections (SC) or monthly intramuscular or subcutaneous injections (M).

Long-term reduction of androgen secretion by repeated or sustained release of LHRH agonists resulting in medical or chemical castration followed by involution of the secondary sex organs has been reported in animal experiments during chronic tolerance studies and confirmed in dose searching studies in preclinical trials for all the listed drugs [8-16].

Table 2. LHRH agonists available for clinical practice

	1	2	3	4	5	6	7	8	9	10	Mode of administration
Natural LHRH	p-GLU	HIS	TRP	SER	TYR	GLY	LEU	ARG	PRO	$GLY\text{-}NH_2$	
1. Bucherelin (Hoechst)	----------					D-SER-(BU^t)	----------			Ethylamide	SC, IN (M)
2. Decapeptyl (Debiopharm)	----------					D-TRP	----------				SC, M
3. Leuprolide (Abbott-Takeda)	----------					D-LEU	----------				SC
4. Nafarelin (Syntex)	----------					D-NAL	----------				IN, SC
5. Zoladex (ICI)	----------					D-SER-(BU^t)	----------			$AZ\text{-}GLY\text{-}NH_2$	M

Phase II Studies

A large number of publications have appeared in the literature on the effect of the various LHRH agonists on patients with prostatic cancer. All these studies were specifically designed to evaluate efficacy and safety of the new treatment. A number of parameters important to the conclusions of these studies are listed in Table 3.

We reviewed a selection of papers where these parameters were reported dealing with a minimum of 50 patients or with a follow up of at least 24 months in patients with metastatic disease. The routes of application together with the different dosages will be presented after analysis of the endocrine and clinical results.

Typical of the serum LH and testosterone (T) fluctuation after LHRH agonist treatment is the steep rise of serum LH followed by a steady decline to basal levels of 2 to 5 mIU/ml with little rise on LH stimulation [17,18]. Follicle stimulating hormone follows a grossly related pattern. Of utmost importance is the subsequent increase in serum T of 4.8 ± 2.2 ng/ml to 5.6 ± 2.4 ng/ml followed by a fall into the castrate range (0.5 ng/ml) after 4 weeks of treatment. This fall correlates with a decrease in serum dihydrotestosterone (DHT) to 18% of its normal levels [18]. The pretreatment values of adrenal androgens, thyroxine, cortisol and prolactin remained unchanged for periods up to 36 months of follow up in some patients [16,17]. Similar results in T suppression to castrate levels were obtained with buserelin [17,18] in 107 and 53 patients, leuprolide [19] in 31 patients with 12 months follow up, decapeptyl [20] in 81 patients and zoladex [21] in 158 patients. The message is that LHRH agonist treatment stimulates T production above normal levels for up to 4 days and results in T castrate levels (a medical castraction) at the end of 4 weeks in all patients. On maintaining the selected drug regimen, no rebound phenomena were observed for periods of up to 48 months of follow up after initiation of treatment.

The different prognostic factors, stage of disease and selection of patients do not allow for comparison of clinical results in all these studies. However, the reported clinical objective remissions according to the European Organisation of Research and

Table 3. Aspects of phase II studies in prostatic cancer

1. Patient characteristics	Number Age Vital status TNMG
2. Statistical characteristics	Eligibility Evaluability
3. Response criteria	Objective Subjective
4. Duration of response	
5. Survival	
6. Side effects - Quality of life	

Table 4. Objective clinical responses in phase II studies

Drug	Ref.	Number	CR-PR (%)	NC (%)	Prog. (%)	Months
Buserelin	[17]	85	52	30	18	48
Decapeptyl	[24]	88	39.6	45.3	15.1	33
Zoladex	[25]	224	59	22	19	47

Reported overall objective responses as complete and partial response (CR-PR), no change or stable disease (NC) and progression (Prog) in the 3 publications with the largest number of patients with long-term follow up in months according to EORTC [17,25] and NPCP [24] criteria.

Treatment of Cancer (EORTC) [22] or to the National Prostatic Cancer Program [23] are presented in Table 4. The reported results indicate that this treatment modality is effective therapy in patients with advanced prostatic cancer. All subjective responses and survival figures reported in these studies are comparable and not one LHRH agonist was reported to be superior to the other analogs in treatment results.

The safety of this treatment has been established by all published studies. No adverse reactions were reported with the inclusion of standard hematological and biochemical tests over long-term periods of observation. The only reported side effects are related to the fluctuations in serum testosterone and its secondary effect on the patient and the biological activity of his hormone-dependent cancer. All patients on questioning reveal loss of libido, impaired erection and subsequent impotence. These side effects are due to the castrate serum levels of T. These secondary effects confirm in a way the pharmacological tolerance of the drug. No studies revealed antibody formation or reported progression of disease with elevated T levels. However, accidental cessation of therapy for up to 12 months may result in a serum T rebound phenomenon, despite the inhibition of spermatogenesis and severe tubular degeneration in the testicles reported in other studies [26,27]. Hot flushes form a part of the expected clinical reaction of the patient to T withdrawal and are reported in approximately 50% of cases [17,18,24,25]. There is a low incidence of breast tenderness.

The clinical reaction to the sudden early rise of serum T is not so clearly related. It has been termed "disease flare-up" in the literature. This vague term refers to the possibility that the initial peak of LH secretion followed by a serum T peak may result in subjective and objective aggravation of symptoms in patients with widespread metastatic disease.

Attention was drawn to the problem by single case reports in the early literature on the subject [28,29], and the knowledge that exogenous testosterone given to patients with prostatic cancer may lead to unfavorable subjective and objective responses [30-33]. Of course, the early flare phenomenon can be caused by disease progression of hormone-independent cancer or by the continued biological growth of hormone-dependent cancers, since LHRH agonist monotherapy takes full effect only after 2 or 3 weeks.

The most frequent subjective response attributed to the flare phenomenon is increased bone pain during the first 4 weeks of therapy. Exacerbation of tumor-related symptoms has been reported in 0-10% of patients in a review of the literature [34]. The biochemical "flare-up" by a related rise in serum acid phosphatase is not always present and sometimes contradictory [17,30]. However, a detailed review of 800 patients treated with LHRH agonist monotherapy versus standard therapy demonstrated a statistically significant worsening of bone pain (4.25% versus 1.5%) during the first month of treatment [35]. A few cases of spinal cord compression or ureteric obstruction were present in both treatment groups. It is self-evident that patients with widespread disease are prone to clinical exacerbation and should be monitored closely in the first weeks of treatment. Most multicenter studies acknowledge the problem and add diethylstilbestrol [36], cyproterone acetate [37], ketoconazole [38] or flutamide [39] to LHRH agonists in the first week of treatment. This simple approach seems to eliminate these unwanted side effects [40]. The routes of application and different doses are presented in Table 5. Local side effects were exceptional and consisted of an occasional rash and, according to the site of application, rhinitis or a local irritation in less than 1% of the patients.

The agonists are not effective when administered orally and the required dose continuity for treatment efficacy demands multiple intranasal applications or daily injections. These are effective but it is obvious that reliable monthly depot formulations with sustained release over long periods of time assure a more complete bioavailability. The pharmaceutical industry developed long-acting preparations such as lactic acid/glycolic acid copolymers (Zoladex) or microcapsule formulations (Decapeptyl). These have been extensively used in clinical studies with efficacy comparable to daily injections or pernasal application. At first developed to improve the convenience of administration and patient compliance, the Zoladex depot formulation proved more efficacious in animal experiments [41] and avoided the LH overstimulation reported with long-term daily injections [42]. It may be concluded that sustained release formulations proved long-term safe control of gonadal steroid secretion in hormone-dependent tumors [43]. The effect of the LHRH agonists depends on the dose used and the regularity of administration.

Phase III Studies

Here a comparison can be made between the new and accepted standard therapy by establishing randomized prospective studies. Several phase III studies comparing LHRH agonist therapy with bilateral orchiectomy or diethylstilbestrol (DES) 3 mg/day

Table 5. Routes of administration and doses of LHRH analogs

Buserelin	subcutaneous injection 3 x 500 ng/day x 7, followed by intranasal insufflation, recommended to give 6 x 100 ng/day in each nostril
Leuprolide	subcutaneous injection 1 mg/day
Decapeptyde	intramuscular injection 3.75 mg/month
Zoladex	subcutaneous injection 3.6 mg/month

Table 6. Percentage of overall response in phase III trials

Author	No.pts.	LHRH agonist	Orch/DES	Follow up (mths)
Swanson [44]	186	86	85	12
Turkes [47]	188	74	79	9
Parmar [46]	104	83	82	12
Emtage* [45]	186	51*	28*	9

* No change/stable disease not included

are listed in Table 6. We selected 4 studies for analysis; each randomized more than 100 patients [44-47].

Garnick coordinated a multicenter study comparing leuprolide 1 mg subcutaneous daily versus DES 3 mg orally per day in untreated patients with advanced prostatic cancer. Time to treatment failure was comparable between the 2 populations. This study involved cross-over therapy after failure of the initial treatment. This blurred the significance of the survival curves. He concludes that the LHRH agonist offers an important alternative to the use of estrogens in the initial treatment of prostatic cancer because of the marked difference in side effects (3% in the leuprolide group vs. 13% in the DES group) [44].

Emtage came to the same conclusion after preliminary analysis of 186 patients with advanced prostatic cancer comparing zoladex 3.6 mg depot with DES 3 mg per day [45]. The overall major complication rate was 1.1% for zoladex-treated patients versus 10.5% for DES-treated patients.

Parmar et al. randomized 104 patients between decapeptyl and bilateral orchiectomy [46]. No differences in response, survival or side effects were reported. A randomized trial coordinated by the Tenovus Institute compared the efficacy of zoladex depot 3.6 mg versus bilateral orchiectomy [47]. The preliminary results reported on 188 patients indicate no differences in treatment response or side effects from the 2 treatments.

Awaiting final analysis over long-term follow up, there is a clear indication that no treatment differences exist between the different LHRH agonists and androgen withdrawal by DES 3 mg/day or bilateral orchiectomy. These results fall in line with the randomized studies performed by the EORTC in patients with prostatic cancer.

Comparisons with DES 3 mg/day vs. cyproterone acetate (CPA) 250 mg daily and medroxyprogesterone acetate (MPA) 500 mg IM twice a week followed by a 200 mg oral dose (EORTC 30761) and the same dose of DES versus estramustine phosphate 280 mg twice daily (EORTC 30762) and bilateral orchiectomy with and without CPA 50 mg tid versus DES 1 mg/day (EORTC 30805) did not demonstrate that any of the hormonal therapies was superior to bilateral orchiectomy [48].

We may conclude that LHRH agonist monotherapy is as effective as any classic hormonal therapy. Its advantages lie with the avoidance of the psychological effect of surgical castration and the total lack of unwanted side effects if the flare-up phenomenon is prevented.

LHRH Agonists as Second-Line Hormonal Therapy

The probability from *in vitro* and *in vivo* animal experiments that LHRH agonists may also act directly on the prostate, prompted the use of leuprolide treatment in patients who progressed after orchiectomy or diethylstilbestrol [49,50]. Of 47 previously treated patients one had a partial response and 15 (32%) had stable disease. Another 25 patients were evaluable for objective response to zoladex treatment in patients who had relapsed after earlier endocrine manipulation [35]. Only one patient showed evidence of partial remission, 20% showed stable disease and the remainder (76%) continued to progress. We may conclude that LHRH agonist therapy is not effective as second-line hormonal therapy.

Indications for LHRH Agonist Treatment

The principal indication of LHRH agonists in patients with advanced prostatic cancer rests primarily with patients who refuse surgical castration. It is of interest to note that the epididymis, conserved in subcapsular orchiectomy, is capable of transferring androgenic steroids, synthesized from the adrenal androgens, to the prostate [51]. There is evidence from the randomized studies that the use of LHRH agonists avoids the cardio-vascular side effects seen after estrogen therapy. Of course, DES 1 mg/day offers an alternative in the absence of cardio-vascular disease [48].

One factor of importance is the possibility of a reversible androgen depletion by LHRH agonists. The aims of a reversible androgen depletion would be [51]:

1. to test response to hormonal therapy in a known carcinoma of the prostate;
2. to test hormonal therapy in a metastatic tumor whose primary source was uncertain.

In primary treatment, if the tumor is hormone sensitive and objective/subjective remission is established, orchiectomy can be used to continue treatment. If progression continues, however, such treatment can be stopped and treatment started with early chemotherapy. The EORTC GU Group prepares protocols to evaluate this approach in patients with advanced prostatic cancer with poor prognostic indicators. This approach may save 20 to 40% of the patients a castration of debatable clinical efficacy.

Conclusions

The development of the LHRH agonists is a major scientific and clinical breakthrough. All phase II studies of preclinical drugs show equal efficacy and a lack of unwanted side effects. They are all comparable in their endocrine responses.

Monotherapy with an LHRH agonist provokes an initial stimulation of serum T production followed by long-term reduction to castration levels. There is a general consensus that this initial stimulation may lead to a flare reaction of disease, especially subjective disease, e.g., bone pain. It is necessary to be cautious with LHRH agonist treatment in patients with widespread metastatic disease and prevention of flare-up with anti-androgens or estrogens is a prudent measure in the first 2 weeks of treatment. Patient compliance, administration of drug and probably superior endocrine control is enhanced with the use of drugs with sustained release. The development of bioavailable lactic acid/glycolic acid copolymers with a 1 to 3-month sustained release is another pharmacological breakthrough.

With equal and proven efficacy in randomized trials of LHRH agonists, bilateral orchiectomy and/or DES 3 mg/day, we may avoid the psychological trauma of surgical castration or the cardiovascular side effects of estrogen treatment in selected cohorts of patients. The utilisation of LHRH agonists as the first treatment to test hormone responsiveness of the tumor system is a novel concept that should be evaluated in clinical research.

REFERENCES

1 Schally AV, Arimura A, Baba Y, Nai RMG, Matsuo H, Redding TW, Debeljuk L: Isolation and properties of the FSH and LH-releasing hormone. Biochem Biophys Res Commun 1971 (43):393-399
2 Labrie F, Bélanger A, Dupont A: LHRH and its Analogues. Basic Clinical Aspects. Excerpta Medica, Amsterdam 1984
3 Redding TW, Schally AV: Inhibition of prostate tumor growth in two rat models by chronic administration of D-Trp analogue of luteinizing hormone-releasing hormone. Proc Natl Acad Sci 1981 (78):6509-6516
4 Sandow J: Pharmacology of LHRH agonists. In: Furr BJA, Wakeling AE (eds) Pharmacology and clinical uses of inhibitors of hormone secretion and action. Baillière Tindall, London 1987 pp 365-384
5 Bhasin S, Swerdloff RS: Mechanisms of gonadotropin-releasing hormone agonist action in the human male. Endocr Rev 1986 (7):106-114
6 Hierowski MT, Altamirano P, Redding TW, Schally AV: The presence of LHRH-like receptors in Dunning R 3327H prostate tumors. FEBS Lett 1983 (154):92-96
7 Vickery BH: Pharmacology of LHRH antagonists. In: Furr BJA, Wakeling AE (eds) Pharmacology and clinical uses of inhibitors of hormone secretion and action. Baillière Tindall, London 1987 pp 385-408
8 Sandow J, von Rechenberg W, Jerzabek G, Engelbart K, Kuhl H, Fraser H: Hypothalamic-pituitary-testicular function in rats after supraphysiological doses of a highly active LRH analogue. Acta Endocrinol 1980 (94):489-497
9 Faure N, Labrie F, Lemay A, Bélanger A, Gourdeau A, Laroc B, Robert G: Inhibition of serum androgen levels by chronic intranasal and subcutaneous administration of a potent luteinizing hormone-releasing hormone (LH-RH) agonist in adult man. Fertility and Sterility 1982 (37):416-424
10 Corbin A: From contraception to cancer: a review of the therapeutic applications of LH-RH analogs as antitumor agents. Yale J Biol Med 1982 (55):27-47
11 Wiegelman W, Solback HG, Kley HK, Kruskemper HL: LH and FSH response to long-term application of an LH-RH analog in normal males. Horm Metab Res 1977 (9):521-522
12 Linde R, Doelle GC, Alexander N, Kirchner F, Vale W, Rivier J, Rabin D: Reversible inhibition of testicular steroidogenesis and spermatogenesis by a potent gonadotropin-releasing hormone agonist in normal men: an approach towards the development of a male contraceptive. N Engl J Med 1981 (305):663-667

13 Vickery BH, McRae GI, Sanders LM, Hoffman P, Pavlou SN: Studies with Nafarelin and a long acting LHRH antagonist. In: Klijn JGM, Paridaens R, Foekens JA (eds) Hormonal Manipulation of Cancer: Peptides, Growth Factors and New (Anti)Steroidal Agents. Raven Press, New York 1987 pp 281-290
14 Vickery BH, McRae GI, Bonash H: Effect of chronic administration of a highly potent LHRH agonist on prostate size and secretory function in geriatric dogs. The Prostate 1982 (3):123-130
15 Dutta AS, Furr BJA, Giles MB, Valcaccia B, Walpole AL: Potent agonist and antagonist analogues of luliberin containing an azaglycine residue in position 10. Biochem and Biophys Res Comm 1978 (81):382
16 Robinson MRG, Denis L, Mahler C, Walker K, Stitch R, Lunglmayr G: An LH-RH analogue (Zoladex) in the management of carcinoma of the prostate: a preliminary report comparing daily subcutaneous injections with monthly depot injections. Eur J Surg Oncol 1985 (11):159-165
17 Jacobi GH, Wenderoth UK, Ehrental W, von Wallenberg H, Spindler HW, Engelmann U, Hohenfellner R: Endocrine and clinical evaluation of 107 patients with advanced prostatic carcinoma under long-term pernasal buserelin or intramuscular decapeptyl depot treatment. In: Klijn JGM, Paridaens R, Foekens JA (eds) Hormonal Manipulation of Cancer: Peptides, Growth Factors and New (Anti)Steroidal Agents. Raven Press, New York 1987 pp 235-248
18 De Jong FH, Schröder FH, Lock MTWT, Debruyne FMJ, de Voogt HJ, Klijn JGM: Effects of long term treatment with the LHRH-analogue buserelin on the pituitary-testicular axis in men with prostatic carcinoma (PCA). In: Klijn JGM, Paridaens R, Foekens JA (eds) Hormonal Manipulation of Cancer: Peptides, Growth Factors and New (Anti)Steroidal Agents. Raven Press, New York 1987 pp 195-202
19 Glode LM, Smith JA Jr, The Leuprolide Study Group: Long-term suppression of luteinizing hormone, follicle-stimulating hormone and testosterone by daily administration of leuprolide. J Urol 1987 (137):57-60
20 Mathé G, Schally AV, Comaru-Schally AM, Mauvernay RY, Vovan ML, Machover D, Misset JL, Court B, Bouchard P, Duchier J, Morin P, Keiling R, Schwarzenberg L, Kerbrat P, Achille E, Tronc JC, Fendler JP, Pappo E, Metz R, Prevot G: Phase II trial with D-Trp-6-LH-RH in prostatic carcinoma: comparison with other hormonal agents. The Prostate 1986 (9):327-342
21 Denis L, Keuppens F, Mahler C, Debruyne FMJ, Weil EHJ, Lunglmayr G, Newling D, Robinson MRG, Richards B, Smith PH, Welan P: Long term therapy with a depot LHRH analogue (Zoladex R) in patients with advanced prostatic cancer. In: Murphy GP, Khoury S, Küss R, Chatelain C, Denis L (eds) Prostate Cancer Part A: Research, Endocrine Treatment and Histopathology. A R Liss, New York 1987 pp 221-227
22 Newling DWW: Criteria for response to treatment of metastatic prostatic cancer. In: Schröder FH, Richards B (eds) Therapeutic principles in metastatic prostatic cancer. A R Liss, New York 1985 pp 205-220
23 Elder JS, Gibbons RP: Results of trials of the USA National Prostatic Cancer Project. In: Schröder FH, Richards B (eds) Therapeutic Principles in Metastatic Prostatic Cancer. A R Liss, New York 1985 pp 221-242
24 Boccardo F: Treatment of advanced prostatic cancer with a long-acting formulation of D-Trp-6 LH-RH. An Italian Prostatic Cancer Project (P.O.N.CA.P.) Study. In: Murphy GP, Khoury S, Küss R, Chatelain C, Denis L (eds) Prostate Cancer Part A: Research, Endocrine Treatment and Histopathology. A R Liss, New York 1987 p 249
25 Debruyne FMJ, Denis L, Lunglmayr G, Mahler C, Newling DWW, Richards B, Robinson MRG, Smith PH, Weil EHJ, Whelan P: Long term therapy with a depot LHRH analogue ("Zoladex") in patients with advanced prostatic carcinoma. J Urol 1987 (in press)
26 Jacobi G: personal communication. 1986
27 Huhtaniemi IT: Testicular changes during GnRH analogue treatment. The Releaser 1986 (1):9-12
28 Faure N, Lemay A, Laroche B, Roberg G, Plante R, Jean C, Thabet M, Roy R, Fazekas ATA: Preliminary results on the clinical efficacy and safety of androgen inhibition by an LHRH agonist alone or combined with an anti-androgen in the treatment of prostatic carcinoma. The Prostate 1983 (4):601-624
29 Kahan A, Delrieu F, Amor B, Cliche R, Steg A: Disease flare induced by D-Trp-6-LHRH analogue in patients with metastatic prostatic cancer. The Lancet 1984:971-972
30 Prout GR, Brewer WR: Response of men with advanced prostatic carcinoma to exogenous administration of testosterone. Cancer 1967 (20):1871-1878
31 Denis LJ, Prout GR Jr, Michielsen JP: Palliative treatment of prostatic cancer with radioactive phosphorus. Excerpta Medica International Congress Series 1976 (178):22-25
32 Fowler JE Jr, Whitmore WF Jr: Considerations for the use of testosterone with systemic chemotherapy in prostatic cancer. Cancer 1982 (49):1373-1377
33 Manni A, Santen RJ, Boucher AE, Lipton A, Harvey H, Simmonds M, White-Hershey D, Gordon RA, Rohner TJ, Drago J, Wettlaufer J, Glode LM: Androgen priming and response to chemotherapy in advanced prostatic cancer. J Urol 1986 (136):1242-1246
34 Denis L, Mahler C: LHRH agonists combination studies. J Endocrinol Invest 1987 (10 Suppl 2):23
35 Milsted RAV: A review of international experience with LHRH agonist "Zoladex" in prostatic carcinoma. J Endocrinol Invest 1987 (10 Suppl 2):18
36 Bouffioux Ch, Denis L, Mahler C, de Leval L: Le traitement du cancer avancé de la prostate au moyen des analogues de la LHRH. Comment prévenir la flambée tumorale (flare-up) initiale possible? Acta Urol Belg 1986 (54):304-308
37 Schröder FH, Lock TMTW, Carpentier PJ, Chadha DR, Debruyne FMJ, de Jong FH, Klijn JGM, Matroos AW, de Voogt HJ: Long term treatment with the LHRH agonist buserelin in metastatic prostatic cancer. Two phase II studies including buserelin plus cyproterone acetate. In: Klijn JGM, Paridaens R, Foekens JA (eds) Hormonal Manipulation of Cancer: Peptides, Growth Factors and New (Anti)Steroidal Agents. Raven Press, New York 1987 pp 225-234

38 Allen JM, Kerle DJ, Ware H: Combined treatment with ketoconazole and luteinizing hormone releasing hormone analogue: a novel approach to resistant progressive prostatic cancer. Br Med J 1983 (287):1766
39 Labrie F, Dupont A, Bélanger A: Complete androgen blockade for the treatment of prostate cancer. In: De Vita VT Jr, Hellman S, Rosenberg SA (eds) Important Advances in Oncology. JB Lippincott Co, Philadelphia 1985 pp 193-205
40 Mahler C, Denis L: Simultaneous administration of a luteinizing hormone releasing hormone agonist and diethylstilbestrol in the initial treatment of prostatic cancer. Abstract Satellite Symposium on Medical Management of Prostate Cancer, Nice, September 2-4, 1987
41 Furr BJA: Treatment of hormone-responsive rat mammary and prostate tumours with "Zoladex" depot. In: Klijn JGM, Paridaens R, Foekens JA (eds) Hormonal Manipulation of Cancer: Peptides, Growth Factors and New (Anti)Steroidal Agents. Raven Press, New York 1987 pp 213-223
42 Williams G, Kerle DJ, Roe SM, Yeo T, Bloom SR: Results obtained in the treatment of prostate cancer patients with Zoladex. In: Schröder FH, Richards B (eds) Therapeutic Principles in Metastatic Prostatic Cancer. A R Liss, New York 1985 pp 287-295
43 Sandow J, Seidel HR, Krauss B, Jerabek-Sandow G: Pharmacokinetics of LHRH agonists in different delivery systems and the relation to endocrine function. In: Klijn JGM, Paridaens R, Foekens JA (eds) Hormonal Manipulation of Cancer: Peptides, Growth Factors and New (Anti)Steroidal Agents. Raven Press, New York 1987 pp 203-212
44 Swanson LJ, Garnick MB: Leuprolide versus diethylstilbestrol for metastatic prostatic cancer. In: Klijn JGM, Paridaens R, Foekens JA (eds) Hormonal Manipulation of Cancer: Peptides, Growth Factors and New (Anti)Steroidal Agents. Raven Press, New York 1987 pp 301-308
45 Emtage LA: A randomized trial comparing Zoladex 3.6 ng depot with Stilbestrol 3 ng/day in advanced prostatic cancer: patient characteristics, reponse and treatment failures. Abstract book ECCO 4, Madrid 1987 p 102
46 Parmar H, Edwards L, Philips RH, Allen L, Lightman SL: Orchiectomy versus long-acting D-Trp-6-LHRH in advanced prostatic cancer. Br J Urol 1987 (59):248-254
47 Turkes AO, Peeling WB, Griffiths K: Treatment of patients with advanced cancer of the prostate: phase III trial, Zoladex against castration. A study of the British Prostate Group. J Endocrin Invest 1987 (10):19 (abstract)
48 Robinson MRG, Hetherington J: The EORTC studies: is there an optimal endocrine management for M1 prostatic disease? World J Urol 1986 (4):171-175
49 Schally AV, Redding TW, Comaru-Scally AM: Potential use of analogs of luteinizing hormone releasing hormones in the treatment of hormone sensitive neoplasms. Cancer Treat Rep 1984 (68):281
50 Sogani PC, Fair WR: Treatment of advanced prostatic cancer. In: Mulholland SG (ed) The Urological Clinics of North America. WB Saunders Co, Philadelphia 1987 pp 353-371
51 Pierrepoint CG, Danès P: A study of the androgenic function of the epididymis. J Steroid Biochem 1984 (20):1105-1111
52 Newling DWW: The value of reversible androgen suppression as a diagnostic test. In: Murphy GP, Khoury S, Küss R, Chatelain C, Denis L (eds) Prostate Cancer Part A: Research, Endocrine Treatment and Histopathology. A R Liss, New York 1987 pp 261-265

Chemical Adrenal Blockade Treatment

L. Denis

Department of Urology, A. Z. Middelheim, Antwerp, Belgium

Bilateral adrenalectomy has been advocated as a second-line endocrine treatment in patients with relapsed prostatic cancer. The rationale of the treatment rests on the resulting decrease in adrenal androgens available to the prostatic cancer cells after first-line androgen withdrawal therapy. Low response rates for short periods of time and morbidity of the procedure led to an active search for agents able to block adrenal androgen steroidogenesis [1,2]. This chapter reviews the clinical results obtained in patients with prostatic cancer with aminoglutethimide, trilostane and ketoconazole.

Adrenal Androgen Biosynthesis

A condensed scheme listing some key steroids in the biosynthesis of androgens and corticosteroids of the adrenal cortex from the uniform cholesterol molecule is presented in Fig 1. The adrenal cortex secretes dihydroepiandrosterone (DHEA) transformed to its sulphate derivative in serum (DHEAS), androstenedione (Δ4-dione)n androst-5-ene 3ß, 17ß-diol (Δ5-diol) and testosterone [3]. All these steroids can be converted into dihydrotestosterone (DHT), the active androgen in prostatic metabolism, in prostatic tissue and other peripheral tissues [4].

In normal men the production of testosterone and Δ4-dione of adrenal origin is very small but the conversion of the other adrenal androgens results in intraprostatic levels of DHT that may be capable of maintaining the stimulation of hormone-dependent cancer cells [5]. This concept has led to the suggestion that more complete therapies of androgen withdrawal, e.g. by elimination of synthesis of adrenal androgens or other interference with molecular androgen stimulation might be more effective than the elimination of testicular androgens only [6]. It should be noted that man is unique among species in producing these amounts of adrenal androgens capable of biological activity.

Aminoglutethimide (AG), trilostane (TS) and especially high doses of ketoconazole (KHD) are capable of blocking the synthesis of adrenal androgens on different levels of the metabolic pathway as shown in Fig. 1 by interference with the P450 enzyme system [7].

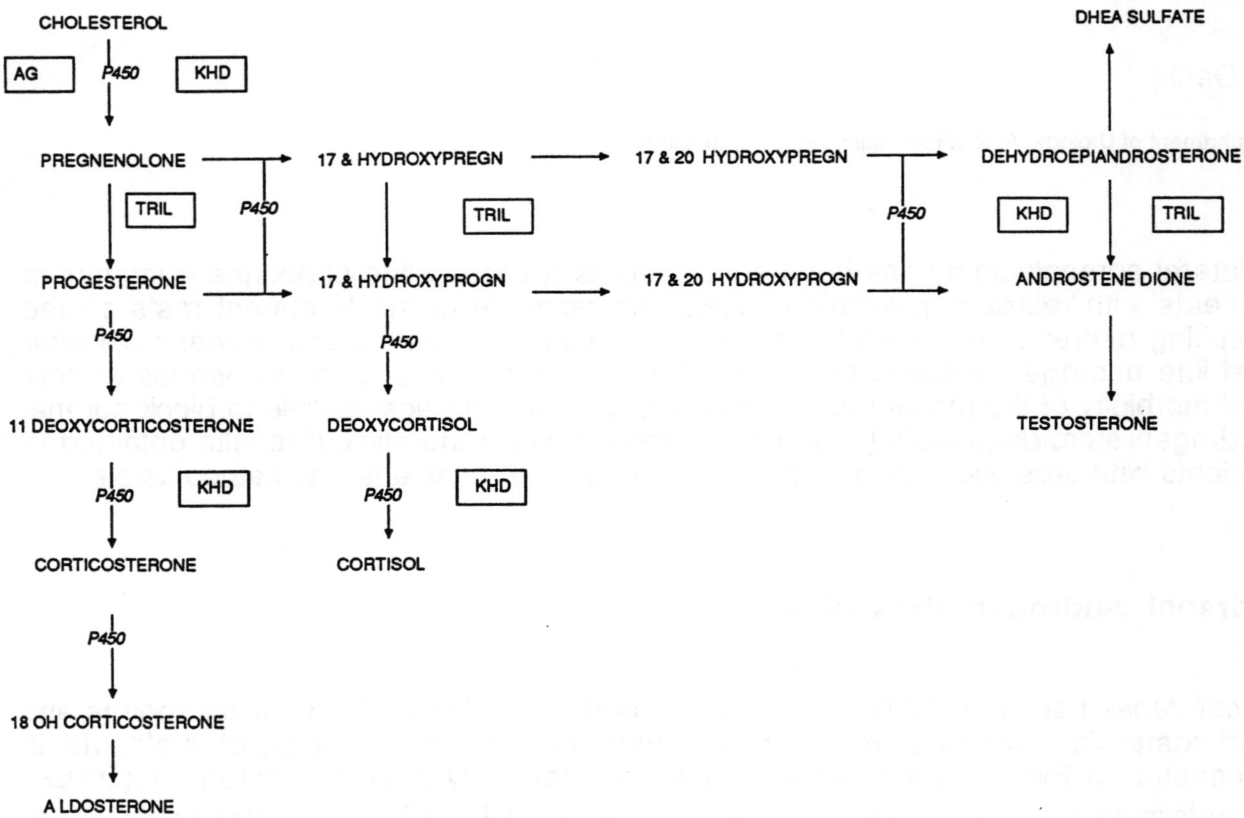

Fig. 1. Simplified scheme of adrenal steroidogenesis and localisation of the blockade by AG, TS and KHD by interference with the P450 enzyme system is indicated.

Aminoglutethimide (3-ethyl-3p aminophenal-2,6-dioxoperidine) (AG)

Aminoglutethimide, a known anti-convulsant drug, provoked adrenal insufficiency in some patients by blocking the transformation of cholesterol into pregnenolone, thus inhibiting the production of aldosterone, cortisol, androgens and estrogens. Other enzymes which can be blocked are the 11-hydroxylase (cortisol formation) and 21-hydroxylase (deoxycortisol formation), but AG is also a potent inhibitor of peripheral aromatase activity. This blocking effect is achieved by binding to the cytochrome P450 moiety of these enzyme complexes [8].

Replacement glucocorticoids are given with AG to avoid cortisol insufficiency and to prevent the reflex rise of adrenocorticotrope hormone (ACTH) which would overcome the results of the chemical blockade.

An active interest in the application of the AG-cortisone therapy in different doses is reflected in several clinical studies in women with metastatic breast cancer [9]. Much less clinical information is available on the AG combination treatment in males with relapsed prostatic cancer. After the initial studies from Robinson [10], a few reports, mainly with subjective response rates, added to clinical experience [7]. At most one third of the patients obtained some benefit for limited periods of time from medical adrenalectomy by AG-cortisone combination. The usual dose of AG was 500 to 1,000 mg/day in divided doses, supplemented by cortisone acetate 2x25 mg/day. The side effects included lethargy, rash and drowsiness in a substantial number of patients. Two Australian studies reported 17 and 21% subjective response in patients with prostatic cancer in relapse, in 126 and 34 patients, respectively, for prolonged periods [11,12]. The exact role of the cortisone supplements related to these results is unknown and further studies with different combinations are warranted [13,14]. Good preliminary results with AG 250 mg tid and hydrocortisone acetate in chronobiological doses of 10 mg at 7 a.m., 5 mg at 3 p.m. and 5 mg at 11 p.m. have been reported as a third-line treatment after castration and relapse following additional anti-androgens or comparable therapies [15]. The blockade of the peripheral aromatization of the androgens to estrogens may play a role in the development and promotion of prostatic cancer [15]. We conclude that aminoglutethimide is an experimental clinical drug with potential applications in metastatic prostatic cancer.

Trilostane (4α,5α,17β)-4,5-epoxy-3,17 d'hydroxyandrost-2.ene.2 carbonitrile (TS)

Trilostane is a synthetic steroid utilised in the treatment of Cushings' disease, low renin hypertension and primary aldosteronism. Its activity depends on the competitive inhibition of the 3ß hydroxysteroid dehydrogenase (see Fig. 1), leading to interference with the androstenedione production in testes and adrenals. However, a concomitant decrease in cortisol synthesis and a rise in DHEA production together with an associated increase in ACTH and luteotropic hormone (LH) in intact males complicate the treatment. The major side effects include gastro-intestinal problems and lethargy [17,18]. We conclude that Trilostane is an experimental drug with no immediate apparent applications in prostatic cancer.

Ketoconazole (Cis-1-acetyl-4 imidazole-1,3 dioxlane-4 piperazine) (K)

Ketoconazole, a synthetic imidazole dioxolane, is active against fungi. This antifungal effect is due to the inhibition of a cytochrome P450 enzyme in fungi at doses of 200 mg daily in men [19]. Higher doses given for periods of time provoked gynecomastia, loss of libido and a dose-related drop in serum testosterone (T) in some patients. These effects were reversible on withdrawal of the drug [2].

The effective blockade of androgen synthesis both by testes and adrenals is due to the fact that high-dose ketoconazole (KHD 400 mg tid) interferes with the cytochrome P450 system of the C17-20 lyase biosynthesis. This provokes a rapid decrease in serum T lasting for 6 to 8 hours and maintained with ketoconazole levels in the serum of 5 ng/ml [21].

<u>Endocrine studies:</u> In 14 previously untreated patients with advanced prostatic cancer, 400 mg KHD was given q 8 hours for at least 2 weeks. Plasma values of DHEA, androstenedione and T dropped by 60 to 80%, with a concomitant rise in hydroxyprogesterone and progesterone. The mean values are presented in Table. 1.

Table 1. Effects of KHD treatment on the main testicular and adrenal steroids in 14 previously untreated patients with metastatic prostate cancer. The results are expressed as mean ± sem.

Plasma levels	Before treatment	After 2 weeks	Student's test on related sample (2 tailed) p values
Testosterone (nmol/l)	15.1 ± 1.3	2.6 ± 0.4	0.0001
Androstenedione (nmol/1)	3.1 ± 0.4	0.6 ± 0.2	0.001
Dehydroepiandrosterone (nmol/l)	6.6 ± 1.0	2.4 ± 0.4	0.0009
17 alpha-hydroxyprogesterone (nmol/l)	2.99 ± 1.09	5.54 ± 0.79	0.04
Progesterone (nmol/l)	1.18 ± 0.09	4.29 ± 0.60	0.0006

The plasma gluco- and mineralcorticosteroids were in general not affected but a discrete rise in 11 deoxycortisol pointed to interference with the 11 hydroxylase system [22]. In one patient a sudden decrease in plasma cortisol contributed to the death of the patient. This observation led to a second study to evaluate basal and stimulated corticosteroid secretion in orchidectomized patients.

KHD, 400 mg tid, was given to 7 castrated patients with prostatic cancer in relapse. Intravenous ACTH stimulation was given on days 0, 14 and 28. Dexamethasone 0.25 mg bid was given together with KHD from day 14 till day 28. KHD alone lowered the basal levels of the androgens (T, androstenedione, DHEA and DHEAS) by 53 to 87% and almost completely inhibited the result of ACTH stimulation at day 14. Progesterone and 17 hydroxyprogesterone levels doubled and elevations were noted for the plasma levels of 11 deoxycortisol, 11 deoxycorticosterone and corticosterone. Aldosterone plasma levels remained unchanged. The basal plasma cortisol levels were slightly lowered but the response to ACTH stimulation was markedly blunted.

After combined KHD dexamethasone treatment the basal and stimulated androgen plasma levels were even more reduced, whereas 11 deoxycortisol, 11 deoxycorticosterone and corticosterone were as low as the plasma cortisol, aldosterone and progesterone profiles were similar as seen under KHD treatment only, but plasma 17 hydroxyprogesterone was markedly increased.

These results show that KHD is able to lower plasma androgen levels in orchidectomized patients and partly blocks the gluco- and mineralocorticoid synthesis even after ACTH stimulation. The addition of dexamethasone corrects not only the impairment of cortisol production but further reduces the plasma androgen levels and lowers the plasma levels of most other precursors [23]. The reflex rise of ACTH in the hypothalamo-pituitary-adrenal axis is able to maintain cortisol plasma levels in most patients but is not strong enough to restore androgen synthesis [24]. Insufficient response in debilitated patients may provoke cortisol insufficiency.

<u>Clinical studies</u>: The clinical results in previously untreated patients parallel the decrease of plasma T by improvement of subjective and objective parameters. A first

multicenter pilot trial noted 95% response, including stable disease in 46 previously untreated patients, 40 of whom were evaluable. Subjective response was noted in 71% of the patients. A second group of 30 patients with relapsed prostatic cancer was followed for 26 ± 16 weeks on KHD. There were 13 patients (46%) with objective responses and 56% with subjective responses.

Subsequent reports provided detailed information to complete the picture on clinical KHD response. A response rate of 88% (objective response, stable disease included), with a follow up of 16 months was reported by Vanuytsel [25]. Twenty-one of the 22 eligible patients showed treatment-related side effects. A steady increase in plasma T to subnormal levels was recorded in some patients after 5 months of treatment. Another 17 previously untreated patients reported by Pont [26] showed similar results. Again, a majority of the patients ceased treatment due to side effects or non-compliance. A small rise in serum T to 100 ng/dl was noted in most patients. Both papers concluded that KHD had limited usefulness as initial therapy.

In a personal series of 20 patients with prostatic cancer in relapse, 8 patients enjoyed a subjective remission, lasting up to 24 months in 2 patients. Not one single objective remission was noted in 15 evaluable patients. All except one died of progressive disease in this period [27]. Identical results (50% subjective improvement and no objective response) were noted by Pont in 11 patients [26]. These results were confirmed by the Dutch South Eastern Urological Cooperative Group in 28 patients with prostatic cancer in relapse: subjective improvement, no objective response and a majority with unwanted side effects [28].

The major side effect of KHD is gastro-intestinal intolerance, which is reported in almost 30% of treated patients, leading to discontinuation of therapy in 10% of patients [29]. A liquid formulation and medication taken during meals may alleviate these symptoms. Clinical symptoms suggestive of adrenal insufficiency have been reported in a few patients as well as a rare case of hepatotoxicity [30].

We conclude that KHD is a remarkable drug leading to more complete androgen withdrawal in untreated patients. However, the reported side effects, the loss of potency, the obligatory 8-hourly intake (because of its pharmacokinetic qualities) and clinical results that only match those obtained with classic therapy, restrict the clinical introduction of this drug. The clinical uses in prostatic cancer are reserved for 2 specific circumstances. Its immediate drop in testosterone biosynthesis makes it an interesting combination for the first 4 days of LHRH treatment to avoid the clinical flare-up caused by the LH stimulation [31], and, maybe more important, the tremendous pain relief obtained in some patients with prostatic cancer in relapse. The extra hormonal mode of action as described by Trachtenberg [32] on prostatic cancer cells by direct cytotoxic effect on cell cultures may play a role. New molecules with more specific P450 activity will be tested in the near future.

REFERENCES

1 Huggins C and Scott W: Bilateral surrenalectomy in prostatic cancer. Ann Surg 1945 (122):1031-1039
2 Blankenstein MA and Bakker GH: Rationale for suppression of adrenal steroidogenesis in advanced prostatic cancer. In: Schröder FH and Richards B (eds) Therapeutic Principles in Metastatic Prostatic Cancer. AR Liss, New York 1985 pp 161-185

3 Labrie F, Poulin R, Simard J, Hubert SF, Spinola P and Marchetti B: Adrenal steroids exert potent estrogenic action in both normal and cancer tissue. In: Klijn JGM (ed) Hormonal Manipulation of Cancer. Raven Press, New York 1987 pp 7-16
4 Harper ME, Pike A, Peeling WB and Griffiths K: Steroids of adrenal origin metabolized by human prostatic tissue both in vivo and in vitro. J Endocrinol 1974 (60):117-125
5 Geller J and Albert J: Effects of castration compared to total androgen blockade on tissue dihydrotesterone (DHT) concentration in benign prostatic hyperplasia (BPH). Urol Res 1987 (15):151-153
6 Labrie F, Dupont A, Belanger A: Complete androgen blockade for the treatment of prostate cancer. In: De Vita, Hellman, Rosenberg (eds) Important Advances in Oncology. Lippincott, Philadelphia 1985 pp 193-217
7 Denis L, Mahler C and De Coster R: Chemical adrenal blockade treatment in prostatic cancer. 1st International Symposium on Advances in Urologic Oncology, San Remo January 22-24, 1987. Acta Medica, Rome p. 61
8 Manni A and Santen RJ: Clinical use of aromatose inhibitors. In: Furr BJA and Wakeling AE (eds) Pharmacology and Clinical Uses of Inhibitors of Hormone Secretion and Action. Bailliere Tindall, London 1987 pp 271-287
9 Klijn JGM: Hormonal Manipulation of Cancer. Raven Press, New York 1987
10 Robinson MRG, Shearer RJ, Fergusson JD: Adrenal suppression in the treatment of carcinoma of the prostate. Br J Urol 1974 (46):555-559
11 Murray R and Pitt P: Aminoglutethimide in the treatment of advanced prostatic cancer. In: Murphy G, Khoury S, Küss R, Chatelain C and Denis L (eds) Prostate Cancer. AR Liss, New York 1987 pp 275-282
12 Harnett PR, Raghavan D, Caterson I, Pearson B, Watt H, Teriana N, Coates A and Coorey G: Aminoglutethimide in advanced prostatic carcinoma. Br J Urol 1987 (59):323-327
13 Plowman PN, Perry LA and Chard T: Androgen suppression by hydrocortisone without aminoglutethimide in orchiectomized men with prostatic cancer. Br J Urol 1987 (59):255-257
14 Fossa SD, Jahnsen JU, Karlsen S, Ogreid P, Haveland H and Trovag A: High-dose medroxyprogesterone acetate versus prednisolone in hormone-resistant prostatic cancer. A pilot study. Eur Urol 1985 (11):11-16
15 Labrie F (1987) Personal communication
16 Stone NN, Laudone VP, Fair WR and Fishman J: Aromatization of androstenedione to estrogen by benign prostatic hyperplasia, prostate cancer and expressed prostatic secretions. Urol Res 1987 (15):165-167
17 Semple CG, Weir SW, Thompson JA, Beastall GH: Trilostane and the normal hypothalamic-pituitary-testicular axis. Clin Endocrinol 1982 (17):99-102
18 Beardwell CG: Clinical uses of trilostane. In: Furr BJA and Wakeling AE (eds) Pharmacology and Clinical Uses of Inhibitors of Hormone Secretion and Action. Bailliere Tindall, London 1986 pp 337-345
19 Van Tyle JH: Ketoconazole. Mechanism of action, spectrum of activity, pharmacokinetics, drug interactions, adverse reactions and therapeutic use. Pharmacotherapy 1984 (4):343-373
20 Pont A, Williams PL, Azhar S, Reitz RE, Bochra Ch, Smith ER and Stevens DA: Ketoconazole blocks testosterone synthesis. Arch Intern Med 1982 (142):2137-2140
21 Vanden Bossche H, Lauwers W, Willemsens G and Cools W: Ketoconazole, an inhibitor of the cytochrome P-450-dependent testosterone synthesis. In: Schröder FH and Richards B (eds) Therapeutic Principles in Metastatic Prostate Cancer. AR Liss, New York 1985 pp 187-196
22 De Coster R and Denis L: High dose ketoconazole therapy blocks testosterone biosynthesis in patients with advanced prostatic cancer: site of actions. Proc XXth Congress of the International Society of Urology, Vienna 1985: 305
23 De Coster R, Mahler C, Denis L, Coene MC and Caers I: Effects of ketoconazole and dexamethasone and ACTH-stimulated adrenal steroidogenesis in orchidectomized prostatic cancer patients. Acta Endocrinol (in press)
24 White MC and Kendall-Taylor R: Adrenal hypofunction in patients taking ketoconazole. Lancet 1985 (i):44-45
25 Vanuytsel L, Ang KK, Vantongelen K, Drochmans A, Baert L and van der Schueren E: Ketoconazole therapy for advanced prostatic cancer: feasibility and treatment results. J Urol 1987 (137):905-908
26 Pont A: Long-term experience with high dose ketoconazole therapy in patients with stage D2 prostatic carcinoma. J Urol 1987 (137):902-904
27 Denis L, Chaban M and Mahler Ch: Clinical applications of ketoconazole in prostatic cancer. In: Schröder FH and Richards B (eds) Therapeutic Principles in Metastatic Prostatic Cancer. AR Liss, New York 1985 pp 319-326
28 Debruyne FMJ, Witjes FA and the Dutch South Eastern Urological Cooperative Group: Ketoconazole HD in the management of hormonally pretreated patients with progressive metastatic disease. In: Murphy GP, Khoury S, Küss R, Chatelain C and Denis L (eds) Prostate Cancer. Part A: Research, Endocrine Treatment and Histopathology. AR Liss, New York 1987 pp 301-313
29 Mahler Ch, Denis L and Chaban M: Ketoconazole in der Behandlung des Prostatakarzinom. In: Hohenfellner R (ed) Verhandlungsberichte der Deutschen Gesellschaft für Urologie. Georg Thieme Velag, Stuttgart 1986 pp 537-538
30 Hay J: Ketoconazole: a reappraisal. Br Med J 1985 (290):260
31 Wenderolt UK and Jacobi GH: Gonadotropin releasing hormone analogues for palliation of carcinoma of the prostate. A new approach to the classical concept. World J Urol 1983 (1):40-48
32 Trachtenberg J and Eichenberger T: Extra hormonal effects of imidazole on human prostatic cancer. J Urol 1987 (137):115A

Total Androgen Blockade

Fritz H. Schröder

Department of Urology, Erasmus University, Rotterdam, The Netherlands

In most Western countries prostatic cancer is the second to third most frequent cause of cancer death in males. The death rate from this tumor has not changed throughout the years. This is mainly due to the fact that most prostatic carcinomas are diagnosed in a metastatic stage. Unfortunately, an effective, curative treatment of this disease is not known [1]. Endocrine management, which produces excellent palliation in 70-80% of all cases, which is associated with an objective response in 20-40% and a significant prolongation of the symptom-free interval, never, or almost never, leads to the cure of a patient. Due to the high incidence of competing causes of death, many patients die with, rather than of, their prostatic carcinoma. Some response rates obtained in recent prospective randomized trials are summarized in Table 1.

The discrepancies in the total response rates are largely due to the consideration of stable disease (SD). It is not felt by most Europeans that SD should be considered a response. Progression-free survival and survival rates with standard treatment (DES 3 mg/day) are in the range of 30% after 1 year and 20% after 5 years [4].

These results are certainly no reason for great optimism and satisfaction with standard management. Progression and death are invariably caused by prostatic cancer becoming hormone unresponsive and killing the patient in spite of endocrine management. The mechanisms leading to hormone-independence of previously hormone-dependent cell populations are poorly understood. Without any doubt, genetic instability of tumor cell populations, combined with the mechanisms of clonal selection and overgrowth determine the biological picture of progression of this disease. It is an open question at this moment whether endocrine manipulation of metastatic prostatic cancer has any impact on the genetic processes leading to hormone independence.

Table 1. Response rates in EORTC protocols 30761 and 30762 (DES 1 mg t.i.d.) and NCPC protocol 500 (DES or castration)

Protocol	Drug	N	CR	PR	SD	Total
EORTC 30761	DES	32	5%	18%	-	23%
EORTC 30762	DES	44	4%	28%	-	32%
NPCP 500	DES or orchiectomy	83	12%	29%	CR+PR=	41%
					40%	81%

Smith et al. 1984 [2], Murphy et al. 1984 [3]

In recent years the approach of total androgen blockade, indicating simultaneous testicular and adrenal suppression, has been strongly advocated by F. Labrie and his group in Canada. This group claims that considerably higher initial response rates, lower progression rates and a smaller chance of transition to the hormone-independent state can be achieved with the combination of an LHRH-agonist or castration combined with a pure anti-androgen as first-line endocrine management [5,6]. Unfortunately, there is much clinical and experimental evidence contradicting this claim, so that uncertainty will persist until the results of well-conducted randomized clinical studies, which compare standard management to total androgen blockade in metastatic cancer patients, become available. Arguments are based on indirect evidence which is interesting in revealing further insights into endocrinological processes connected with prostatic carcinoma, but which, unfortunately, is not conclusive in either direction. Some of this evidence will be reviewed, realizing that within a few years definitive clinical answers will have been obtained which will make this report irrelevant.

Model Systems

Animal and *in vitro* model systems have greatly contributed to our understanding of malignant growth and its regulation. The applicability of these systems to the human situation is, however, usually quite limited. It is necessary to characterize such systems carefully, in order to identify similarities with the human tumor to be studied. Only if a close relation can be established concerning certain features of model systems with human tumors, can a relevant answer be expected out of experimental work with such systems.

Unfortunately, only very few experimental prostatic tumors that grow in animals are available for studying the endocrine dependence of this disease. It will be impossible to review, within this context, the animal models available for human prostatic carcinoma. Such a review has recently been presented by Romijn et al. [7]. On the other hand, the 3 major model systems, the Dunning R-3327 Copenhagen rat tumor line, the Noble rat tumor line and the transplanted lines in the nude mouse, namely the PC-82 line, offer much insight into the mechanisms of endocrine dependence and hormone unresponsiveness. These models also show the extreme variability of the biological features related to endocrine dependence, which becomes even more exaggerated if the androgen-dependent Shionogi mouse mammary tumor [8] is also considered. Table 2 summarizes some of the important characteristics of these models.

It is remarkable that all these models have different properties as far as their pathology, their rate of growth and their endocrine dependence is concerned. Maximal suppression of growth of the hormone-dependent fraction is usually obtained by castration; elimination of adrenal androgens does not have any additional effect, except in the Shionogi tumor. The Noble rat tumor is inducible in the dorsal prostate of the Noble rat by chronic stimulation with estrogens. Conversion from estrogen dependence to androgen dependence is seen and can be manipulated. Substitution of the animals with low doses of the stimulating hormone prevents the transition to autonomous growth. Complete withdrawal of estrogens or androgens will lead to

Table 2. Some properties of animal model systems for human prostatic carcinoma

	Dunning R3327 [9]	Noble rat tumor [10]	PC-82 [11] (nude mouse)	Shionogi tumor[8]
Origin	Copenhagen rat	NB rat, dorsal	human	
Adeno-	mouse mammary	prostate	carcinoma	carcinoma
Histology	adenocarcinoma, variable, undifferentiated lines	variable, adenocarcinoma + solid carcinoma	adenocarcinoma cribriform	adenocarcinoma
Metastases	yes, bone, lungs, nodes	lung (30%)	no	-
Sublines	yes (H,HI,AT and others	yes, androgen- and estrogen-dependent, autonomous	no	yes, by in-vitro cloning
Hormone-dependence	yes, independent sublines due to genetic instability and clonal selection	progress to autonomy is dependent on endocrine manipulations	androgen-dependent, no autonomous growth	androgen-dependent, variable, autonomous lines autonomy prevented by anti-androgen [12]
Growth rate (doubling time in days)	2-20	4-6	16	1
Growth in vitro	yes	?	short term	yes

autonomous growth of the previously estrogen- or androgen-dependent sublines.

The only way of directly investigating the hormone dependence of human prostatic carcinoma in an experimental system *in vivo* is by means of heterotransplantation into immunosuppressed animals or nude mice. The nude mouse model has led to the origination of at least 6 permanent lines, 3 of which were originated in the laboratory of the Department of Urology, Erasmus University, Rotterdam (The Netherlands). The PC-82 line is the best characterized. The tumor is completely hormone-dependent, no autonomous growth results after prolonged cultivation or after castration. Growth is arrested if plasma testosterone drops below 1 ng/ml. Growth arrest is also found to be associated with tissue levels of DHT ranging from 3.4-4.2 ng/g tissue [13]. These levels are high and just below the DHT levels that are found in human prostatic carcinoma tissue in intact, non-castrated patients.

The Shionogi tumor *in vitro* is much more sensitive to androgens. Labrie and Veilleux [12] have, by single cell plating, identified clones of cells that are extremely sensitive to androgen stimulation. Stimulation of 10 different clones of Shionogi cells by DHT *in vitro* were seen at concentrations ranging from 10^{-8} -10^{-11} molar. This unique behavior is not seen in any of the other hormone-dependent tumor models and there is very little evidence that human prostatic carcinoma *in vivo* behaves in the described way. It has also been stated that the transition of the Shionogi tumor cells to the autonomous state can be prevented by total androgen blockade by means of the anti-androgen flutamide [5]. This observation has not been reproduced in any of the other model systems. On the contrary, total withdrawal of the inducing hormone will promote autonomous growth in the Noble tumor model.

To summarize this section on models for prostatic carcinoma, it is stressed once again that there seems to be great variability in the characteristics of animal models for endocrine-dependent tumors. The fact that one of these models, the Shionogi tumor, responds *in vitro* to extremely low DHT concentrations with a growth response, and that in this particular model the transition to the hormone-independent state can be inhibited by total androgen withdrawal, is not indicative of the behavior of endocrine-dependent tumor cells in general or of the behavior of human prostatic carcinoma in patients. On the other hand, the extreme variability of endocrine dependence seen in animal models does not exclude the possibility that human prostatic carcinoma may also be very variable in its response to endocrine management.

Observations in Human Males

After castration of an intact human male, plasma testosterone levels decrease to about one tenth of the normal value, namely from 5.8 ng/ml to less than 0.58 ng/ml. At our own institution, the range of normal plasma testosterone values was found to be 2.8-14.0 ng/ml. It is thought that the remaining plasma testosterone originates from peripheral metabolization of the 3 adrenal androgens dihydro-epi-androsterone (DHEA), dihydro-epi-androsterone sulphate (DHEAS) and androstene-dione. DHEA is the most important of these. The most important intra-prostatic androgen is dihydrotestosterone (DHT). The prostate itself (and several other tissues) can metabolize adrenal androgens and testosterone to DHT, and the DHT level in the prostatic tissue is probably the most relevant parameter for the amount of androgenic stimulation present at a given time.

It has been shown by Geller [14,15] and his coworkers that testosterone levels in prostatic carcinoma drop to about one half of the pre-operative levels after castration and to about twice the level found in non-target tissues. These data are summarized in Table 3.

Table 3. Levels of 5 dihydrotestosterone (DHT) in human prostatic tissues

Tissue type	No.pts.	DHT (ng/g, x and range)
Normal prostate	6	x = 2.1 (0.7 - 3.0)
BPH	16	x = 5.0 (2.5 - 9.3)
Ca. prostate	17	x = 3.2 (1.0 - 6.6)
Ca. prostate after castration	3	x = 1.6 (1.2 - 2.3)
Ca. under DES treatment	4	x = 3.38 (0.2 - 4.4)
Non target tissue	15	x = 0.8 (0.2 - 2.4)

Geller 1978, 1984 [14,15]

There is little doubt that the relatively high tissue DHT levels found after castration are sustained by adrenal androgens. This shows the capability of the prostate to concentrate androgens to produce DHT concentrations in the range of 2 ng/g tissue. Such levels of DHT will stimulate several androgen-dependent biological systems, such as the ventral prostrate of the rat and certainly the extremely androgen-sensitive clones of the Shionogi tumor. The big question is whether they have any biological importance in stimulating the growth of human prostatic carcinoma after castration. It has been shown by Labrie and coworkers that, with the application of total androgen blockade by means of an LHRH-agonist combined with the anti-androgen flutamide, it is possible to decrease DHT concentrations in prostatic cancer tissue to approximately 0.2 ng of free DHT per gram of tissue [16]. Is it necessary for growth suppression of human prostatic carcinoma to reduce tissue DHT to such low levels? As mentioned in the introduction, only good clinical trials will answer this question. In the meantime the field is open for discussion.

There is much biological and clinical evidence that the function of human accessory sex organs is dependent on a normal testicular androgen production and that adrenal androgens are insufficient to support their function. Pre-puberal castration leads to prostatic atrophy. The development of secondary sexual characteristics such as the growth of pubic hair, the growth of the penis and the deepening of the male voice are dependent on the presence of intact testicular function. After castration erectile failure and loss of libido result and the secretional function of sexual glands is arrested and not restored by adrenal androgens. In a retrospective study of autopsy cases, Oesterling et al. [17] have compared the morphology of prostates in 3 distinct groups. Four men had suffered from panhypopituitarism and had never exhibited any adrenal or testicular function, nor were they substituted with any steroid hormones. A second group of 4 men had normal adrenal glands but no testicular function or androgen substitution at any period during their lifetime. Eight normal age-matched males with intact testicles served as control. Morphometrical findings obtained from histological slides of the prostates of these cases were compared for epithelial height, acinar area, acinar diameter and epithelial height:nuclear height ratio. All parameters showed a highly significant difference between group 1 and 2 and the control group, respectively. No differences were seen between the patients suffering from panhypopituitarism and those suffering from lack of testicular endocrine function. This clearly indicates that adrenal androgens are not capable of maintaining the normal function and morphological expression of the human prostate. Again, this represents only indirect evidence, the possibility that prostate *cancer* cells behave differently cannot be excluded.

Results of Clinical Trials

Since 1982 the group of Canadian investigators associated with Labrie have claimed that total androgen suppression in the primary management of human prostatic carcinoma is a better treatment than castration or other standard forms of management. This claim is based on phase II information resulting from trials that use weak response criteria to identify what is called a "positive objective response". The most recent communication describes a prospective multicenter study of 94 patients with histologically proven stage D2 prostatic adenocarcinoma [5] treated by castration or by LHRH-agonist plus pure anti-androgen. The castration arm was discontinued when 4 of the 7 patients entered to this arm died after 11.5, 16, 17 and 29 months. The group of 87 patients who received the combined treatment were shown to have an initial response rate of 100% and a probability of a continuing positive response at 2 years of 81%. Of the 8 patients (11.9%) who relapsed, one died of prostatic carcinoma and 3 of other causes. This compares extremely favorably with the data shown above in which standard treatment of similar patients is followed by progression in approximately 30% within 1 year. In the study of Labrie et al. [5], however, the average observation time for the whole group of patients is only 16.2 months. Recruitment to both arms certainly is not equal and one wonders about the selection of patients.

The clinical studies carried out by the Canadian group can be criticized in relation to the use of response criteria that are considered by many to be weak, the obviously inaccurate randomization in the prospective study just mentioned [5], the fact that the patients reported must be selected from a much larger group (what are the selection criteria?), the inadequate description of selection criteria and of the characteristics of patients at entry. Still, the controversy remains and will only be solved by a large, well-conducted and completed randomized clinical study of patients with metastatic prostatic carcinoma, which compares standard treatment to a regimen of total androgen suppression.

In reviewing the recent literature, some information strongly seems to contradict Labrie's findings and hypotheses. Prospective randomized studies reported by Brisset and co-workers [18] and Navratil [19], compared standard regimens to total androgen suppression using an LHRH analog (buserelin) in combination with anandron, a potent pure anti-androgen. In spite of some suggestions that there may be a slight disadvantage for the regimen of total androgen blockade in the early response rates, the study showed no significant advantage as far as the progression rates were concerned.

Protocol 30805 of the EORTC-GU Group compares castration alone to castration combined with 150 mg of cyproterone-acetate per day and to 1 mg of DES per day in a prospective randomized trial of patients with metastatic prostatic carcinoma; this trial started in 1980. The dose of DES (1mg/day) is of some interest since Shearer et al. [20] have shown that this dose does not reduce plasma testosterone to castration levels. Averages remain in the range of 0.8-1.0 ng/ml. The study thus compares castration as standard treatment to a regimen that lowers plasma testosterone to about 2 times castration level and to a regimen of total androgen suppression. During the first evaluation carried out 1 year after termination of the trial, it became evident that neither progression nor survival rates showed any differences between the 3 treatment groups. Seventy-nine patients were treated by orchiectomy and 32 failed. Eighty-two patients were treated by orchiectomy plus CPA and 33 failed. Of 80 patients treated by DES 1 mg/day 30 patients failed. The Kaplan-Maier curves are superimposable.

Extensive discussion has resulted as to the point whether cyproterone-acetate is as potent and effective an anti-androgen as flutamide. A considerable volume of literature has accumulated on this subject, of which only 4 papers are included in this list of references [23,24,25,26]. The author's own standpoint is in agreement with a letter published in Lancet in 1985 [26]. Plasma testosterone levels and acid phosphatase activity determined by an immunochemical assay were compared in frequent

determinations during the first 2 weeks of management in 13 patients treated with buserelin and cyproterone-acetate and in 12 patients treated with buserelin alone. Cyproterone-acetate given in a dosage of 150 mg per day was not capable of counteracting the initial rise in plasma testosterone resulting from buserelin treatment during the first 2 weeks with a top after 3-6 days. During the same time, however, namely on days 3 and 6, prostatic acid phosphatase already had come down in the group treated with cyproterone-acetate in addition to buserelin. In the patients treated with buserelin alone a sharp rise of acid phosphatase occurred during the same period of time. This clearly shows that in the clinical situation cyproterone-acetate acts as an anti-androgen in spite of rising plasma testosterone by decreasing a parameter for tumor mass, prostatic acid phosphatase. This matter is discussed further in the chapter on anti-androgens in this Monograph. The EORTC Genito-Urinary Group is presently conducting 2 phase III randomized prospective trials that are designed to give decisive answers to these open questions. In the 2 protocols, previously untreated patients with metastatic prostatic cancer are randomized as follows:
Protocol 30843: Buserelin (LHRH agonist) 1200 µg/day plus cyproterone acetate (CPA) 150 mg/day versus buserelin 1200 µg/day plus CPA 150 mg during the first 2 weeks versus castration.
Protocol 30853: Depot zoladex (LHRH agonist) plus flutamide 750 mg versus castration.

The endpoint of both studies is progression and patients are followed to death for evaluation of survival. These studies should assist in the continuing evaluation of the concept of total androgen blockade and of the most effective hormonal treatment of metastatic prostatic cancer.

REFERENCES

1 Whitmore WF: The natural history of prostatic cancer. Cancer 1973 (32):1104-1112
2 Smith PH, Pavone Macaluso M, Viggiano G, De Voogt HJ, Lardennois B, Robinson MRG, Richards B: EORTC protocols in prostatic cancer. In: Denis L, Murphy GP, Prout GR, Schröder FH (eds) Controlled Clinical Trials in Urologic Oncology. Raven Press, New York 1984 pp 107-111
3 Murphy GP, Slack NH and participants in the National Prostatic Cancer Project: Current status of the National Prostatic Cancer Project treatment protocols. In: Denis L, Murphy GP, Prout GR, Schröder FH (eds) Controlled Clinical Trials in Urologic Oncology. Raven Press, New York 1984 pp 119-134
4 Smith PH, Suciu S, Robinson MRG, Richards B, Bastable JRG, Glashan RW, Bouffioux C, Lardennois B, Williams RE, De Pauw M, Sylvester R: A comparison of the effect of Diethylstilbestrol with low dose estramustine phosphatase in the treatment of advanced prostatic cancer: final analysis of a phase III trial of the European Organization for Research on the Treatment of Cancer. J Urol 1986 (136):619-623
5 Labrie F, Dupont A, Belanger A, Giguere M, Lacoursiere Y, Edmon J, Monfette G, Bergeron V: Combination therapy with Flutamide and castration (LHRH agonist or orchiectomy) in advanced prostate cancer: a marked improvement in response and survival. J Steroid Biochem 1985 (23):833-841
6 Labrie F, Dupont A, Belanger A: Complete androgen blockade for the treatment of prostate cancer. In: DeVita Jr VT, Hellman S, Rosenberg SA (eds) Important Advances in Oncology 1985. JB Lippincott Company, Philadelphia 1985 pp 193-217
7 Romijn JC, Van Steenbrugge GJ, Blankenstein MA, Schröder FH: Animal models in prostatic cancer. In: Pavone-Macaluso M, Smith PH (eds) Cancer of the Prostate and Kidney. Plenum Press, New York and London 1983 pp 35-44
8 Matsumoto K, Sato B, Kitamura Y: Roles of androgen and its receptors in mouse mammary tumor. In: Leung S (ed) Hormonal Regulation of Mammary Tumors. Vol IB. Eden Press, Montreal 1982 pp 216-244
9 Isaacs JT, Heston WDW, Weissman RM, Coffey DS: Animal models of the hormone-sensitive and insensitive prostatic adenocarcinomas, Dunning R3327-H, R3327-HI and R3327-AT. Cancer Res 1978 (38):4353-4359
10 Noble RL: The development of prostatic adenocarcinoma in the NB rats following prolonged sex hormone administration. Cancer Res 1977 (17):1929

11 Van Steenbrugge GJ, Groen M, Romijn JC, Schröder FH: Biological effects of hormonal treatment regimens on a transplantable human prostatic tumor line (PC-82). J Urol 1984 (131):812-817
12 Labrie F, Veilleux R: A wide range of sensitivities to androgens develops in cloned Shionogi mouse mammary tumor cells. The Prostate 1986 (8):293-300
13 Van Steenbrugge GJ, Van Dongen JJW, Reuvers PJ, De Jong FH, Schröder FH: Transplantable human prostatic carcinoma (PC-82) in athymic nude mice: I. Hormone dependence and the concentration of androgens in plasma and tumor tissue. Submitted for publication
14 Geller J, Albert J, Loza D, Geller S, Stoeltzing W, De La Vega D: DHT concentrations in human prostate cancer tissue. J Clin Endocrinol Metab 1978 (46):440
15 Geller J, Albert JD, Nachtsheim DA, Loza D: Comparison of prostatic cancer tissue dihydrotestosterone levels at the time of relapse following orchiectomy or estrogen therapy. J Urol 1984 (132):693-696
16 Labrie F, Luthy I, Veilleux R, Simard J, Belanger A, Dupont A: New concepts on the androgen sensitivity of prostate cancer. In: Murphy GP (ed) Second International Symposium on Prostate Cancer. Alan R Liss, New York 1987 (in press)
17 Oesterling JE, Epstein JI, Walsh PC: The inability of adrenal androgens to stimulate the adult human prostate: an autopsy evaluation of men with hypogonadotropic hypogonadism and panhypopituitarism. J Urol 1986 (136):1030-1034
18 Brisset JM, Boccon-Gibod L, Botto H, Camey M, Cariou G, Duclos JM, Duval F, Gonties D, Jorest R, Lamy L, Le Duc A, Moutin A, Petit M, Prawerman A, Richard F, Savatovsky I, Vallancien G: Anandron (RU 23908) associated to surgical castration in previously untreated stage D prostate cancer: a multicenter comparative study of two doses of the drug and of a placebo. In: Khoury S, Murphy GP (eds) Cancer of the Prostate. Alan R Liss, New York 1987 (in press)
19 Navratil H: Double-blind study of anandron versus placebo in stage D2 prostate cancer patients receiving Buserelin. Results on 49 cases from a multicenter study. In: Khoury S, Murphy GP (eds) Cancer of the Prostate. Alan R Liss, New York 1987 (in press)
20 Shearer RJ, Hendry WF, Sommerville IF, Fergusson JD: Plasma testosterone: an accurate monitor of hormone treatment in prostatic cancer. Br J Urol 1973 (45):668-677
21 Robinson MRG, Hetherington J: The EORTC studies: is there an optimal endocrine management for M1 prostatic cancer? World J Urol 1986 (4):1-5
22 Poyet P, Labrie F: Comparison of the antiandrogen/androgenic activities of flutamide, cyproterone acetate and megestrol acetate. Mol Cell Endocrinol 1985 (42):283-288
23 Knuth UA, Hano R, Nieschlag E: Effect of flutamide or cyproterone acetate on pituitary and testicular hormones in normal men. J Clin Endocrinol Metab 1984 (59):963-969
24 Habenicht UF, Witthaus E, Neumann F: Antiandrogene und LH-RH-Agonisten; Endokrinologie in der Initialphase ihrer Anwendung. Akt Urol 1986 (17):10-16
25 Huang JK, Bartsch W, Voigt KD: Interactions of an anti-androgen (cyproterone acetate) with the androgen receptor system and its biological action in the rat ventral prostrate. Acta Endocrinol 1985 (109):569-576
26 Klijn JGM, De Voogt HJ, Schröder FH, De Jong FH: Combined treatment with Buserelin and Cyproterone acetate in metastatic prostatic carcinoma. Lancet 1985 (31):493

Second-Line Endocrine Treatment

G.H. Jacobi

Urologische Klinik und Poliklinik, Johannes Gutenberg Universität, Mainz, Germany

It was a milestone of cancer therapy in general when Huggins et al. [1] in 1941 first reported the beneficial clinical effects of bilateral orchiectomy in patients with prostate cancer, and the use of castration or estrogens as standard therapy remained the first-line treatment for many years. It was furthermore the beginning of a development which, over the following decades, led to the manipulation of testicular androgen synthesis and to attempts to eliminate other possible sources of male hormones.

However, within 4 years the same author recognised that, despite androgen withdrawal, relapses occurred in some of the patients treated and that patients still died from cancer after an initial good response. Knowing that the adrenal gland produces steroids with androgenic potency, Huggins and Scott [2] advocated elimination of this hormonal source by bilateral adrenalectomy. Strictly speaking, this must be considered as the introduction of the so-called 'total androgen blockade', for which others are claiming credit 40 years later (see chapter 8). Adrenalectomy, however, provided short-term benefit only in some patients and it was Scott again who asked himself the question: "What makes the prostate grow?", when he introduced hypophysectomy as the final step of hormone deprivation [3]. Years later it became possible to block adrenal hormone synthesis pharmacologically [4], but further research showed that in patients who relapsed after castration as *first-line* treatment neither peripheral testosterone [5], testosterone in the adrenal venous blood [6], nor androgenic adrenal metabolites (androstenedione, DHEA) were elevated [7]. Since adrenalectomy and hypophysectomy produced a beneficial response rate akin to that of a placebo effect, they were soon abandoned. Nevertheless, modern pharmacology has made possible the development of compounds which can be used to manipulate the hormone milieu for *second-line* treatment or in order to replace the conventional standard therapy.

Rationale for Second-Line Treatment

In recent years the standard hormone regimens have been supplanted by antiandrogens or LHRH analogues as first-line treatment, since both are more easily accepted by the patient. Therefore, second-line treatment must be related to the degree of androgen deprivation provided by the initial hormone manipulation.

If we define second-line treatment as: any contrasexual measure given to patients who have failed primary hormonal treatment whose aim was to lower the levels of peripheral androgens or to block their action at the tumour, then some logical options become apparent.

Example 1: Primary estrogen has not achieved androgen suppression into the castrate range ---> orchiectomy as second line.

Example 2: Primary flutamide treatment (see chapter 5 for pure antiandrogens) failed ---> orchiectomy or LHRH analogues for androgen withdrawal as second line.

Other possibilities must essentially be based on the hypothesis of adrenal steroids being significant growth factors (chapter 8).

Example 3: Primary castration or LHRH analogues failed ---> intraprostatic blocking of androgens from adrenal origin by antiandrogen.

Example 4: Primary castration or LHRH analogues failed ---> suppression of adrenal steroid synthesis by aminoglutethimide.

There are also sequential treatment strategies which are sometimes used in practice but which lack a scientific rationale.

Example 5: Secondary LHRH analogues cannot do more therapeutically when primary castration failed, and vice versa.

Compounds and Literature Review

Table 1 lists the theoretical possibilities, some historical, some in clinical use and others still investigational. Since exact criteria for the diagnosis of relapse (i.e., progression) are used only in prospective studies, reports of meaningful interpretations are rare.

Stone et al. [8] studied 30 patients who progressed whilst on treatment with stilbestrol, dienestrol, cyproterone acetate or orchiectomy. Objective evidence of relapse was based on bone scan, X-ray, lymphadenectomy or serum acid phosphatase (PAP), the bone scan being the most useful criterion. Of the 21 patients submitted to orchiectomy as second line, only 1 patient developed objective regression and only 3 patients improved subjectively. It is conceivable that the first-line treatment had caused androgen suppression.

Fossa et al. [9] investigated 24 patients who failed to show suppression of plasma testosterone to less than 3 nmol/l plasma. Strict response criteria were used and medroxyprogesterone acetate (1 g/day) was given as second-line regimen. There were 8 remissions (mainly subjective!) which lasted only 4 months on average. Gestonorone caproate, another progestational agent, was investigated at our institution. Eighteen patients with painful metastatic disease with objective relapse after orchiectomy were treated with 400 mg/week i.m. There were no objective responders. Three patients showed pain relief, 2 a decrease in serum acid phosphatase, and all patients needed other palliative measures. In another study of a comparable patient selection, 63 patients were treated with high doses of stilphostrol by intravenous infusion of 1.2 g/day over 10 days and orally thereafter. This treatment

Table 1. Options for second-line hormone manipulation

Treatment	Value	Cross references
Stilbestrol	historical	chapters 4,11
Estramustine phosphate	in use	chapters 4,10
Stilphostrol (high dose)	in use	
Progestins	in use	
Antiandrogens	in use	chapter 5
Androgen synthesis suppressors (enzyme blockers)	investigational	
Adrenalectomy	historical	chapter 7
Adrenal inhibitors	investigational	chapter 7
Hypophysectomy	historical	
LHRH analogues alone	in use	chapter 6
Orchiectomy	in use	chapters 3,11
Total androgen blockade	investigational	chapter 8

showed very encouraging palliative effects: pain relief (62%), improved upper urinary tract (26%), decreased PAP (45%).

However, palliation lasted only for 3-12 months. Almost identical subjective responses with this estrogen preparation have been reported by Van Erps et al. [10]. It has been suggested that stilphostrol will concentrate in areas of metastases which contain high levels of acid phosphatase, allowing active stilbestrol to act directly upon the tumour cell. There is, however, a certain cardiovascular toxicity and sudden cardiac deaths have been seen.

Final Comment

If the conclusions drawn from early experiences with secondary adrenalectomy and hypophysectomy are correct, if our knowledge on the metabolism of adrenal steroids in healthy men is also valid for the prostate cancer patient, and if preliminary data of still ongoing studies with total androgen blockade prove valid, there should be no scientific rationale for second-line hormone treatment, once castrate levels of testosterone have been achieved by the first-line regimen. This simple logical view is, however, not completely supported by the literature as certain clinical reports (some anecdotical in nature) demonstrate evidence of responses. It seems certain that our understanding of all aspects of the endocrine control of prostate cancer is not yet complete.

REFERENCES

1 Huggins C, Stevens Jr RE, Hodges CV: Studies on prostatic cancer: effects of castration on advanced carcinoma of prostate gland. Arch Surg 1941 (43):209-223

2 Huggins C, Scott WW: Bilateral adrenalectomy in prostatic cancer. Clinical features and urinary excretion of 17-ketosteroids and estrogen. Ann Surg 1945 (122):1031-1041

3 Scott WW: Endocrine management of disseminated prostate cancer, including bilateral adrenalectomy and hypophysectomy. Trans Am Ass GU Surg 1953 (44):101-104

4 Hughes SWM, Burley DM: Aminoglutethimide: a 'side effect' turned to a therapeutic advantage. Postgrad Med J 1970 (46):409-417

5 Mackler MA, Liberti JP, Smith MJV, Koontz WW, Prout GR: The effect of orchiectomy and various doses of stilbestrol on plasma testosterone levels in patients with carcinoma of the prostate. Invest Urol 1972 (9):423-425

6 Sanford EJ, Paulson DF, Rohner Jr TJ, Santen RJ, Bardin CW: The effects of castration on adrenal testosterone secretion in men with prostatic carcinoma. J Urol 1977 (118):1019-1021

7 Walsh PC: Physiologic basis for hormonal therapy in carcinoma of the prostate. Urol Clin North Am 1975 (2):125-140

8 Stone AR, Hargreave TB, Chisholm GD: The diagnosis of oestrogen escape and the role of secondary orchiectomy in prostatic cancer. Br J Urol 1980 (52):535-538

9 Fossa SD, Jahnsen JU, Karlsen S, Ogreid P, Haveland H, Trovag A: High-dose medroxyprogesterone acetate versus prednisolone in hormone-resistant prostatic cancer. Eur Urol 1985 (11):11-16

10 Van Erps P, Denis L, Nowé P, Keuppens F: Diethylstilbestrol diphosphate in the treatment of prostatic cancer in relapse. In: Denis L, Murphy GP, Prout GR, Schröder FH (eds) Controlled Clinical Trials in Urologic Oncology. Raven Press, New York 1984

Chemotherapy

A.T. van Oosterom

Department of Oncology, University Hospital, Antwerp, Belgium

The median age of patients with prostatic cancer is high and patients with advanced metastatic prostatic cancer are therefore even older. However, the decision to use chemotherapy must entail a consideration of the balance between likely benefits and expected toxic effects of the therapy. In chemocurable diseases in younger patients the decision is easy. In most other adult malignancies it is more difficult, as has recently been discussed by Kearsley [1]. He stressed the need for the therapist to be realistic in his aim of palliation. Particular attention has to be paid to the impact of the induced toxicities to the patients, together with the impact of investigations used in trying to assess response. These remarks are even more important for the physician treating these elderly prostatic cancer patients.

Conflicting opinions concerning the role of chemotherapy have recently come from Murphy [2], who stated in 1984 that it is effective, whilst Eisenberger et al. [3] of the N.C.I., Bethesda, U.S.A., felt that the role of non-hormonal cytotoxic chemotherapy has not been established.

The 2 main problems are the biological behaviour of carcinoma of the prostate, which can be characterised by a number of different biological patterns and the different response assessment methods used in the literature. Firstly the different biological patterns: prostatic cancer exhibits a wide spectrum of natural history from a virulent life-threatening disease to one which is almost 'benign' and may not inconvenience the patient at all. Depending upon the tumour kinetics and pathology, the cancer may remain localised to the prostate or spread either by the lymphatic route to the pelvic lymph nodes and from there to the skeleton, or directly by the haematogenous route mainly to the axial skeleton. More than 50% of the patients with prostate cancer present with metastatic disease predominantly in bone. Some suggest a fourth variety of disease: patients developing soft tissue or visceral lesions as well. This group of patients has a much poorer outlook than the others. The second problem in evaluating chemotherapy is the different definitions of response applied in the various study groups. This problem is compounded by the small numbers of patients in many studies. The differences in opinion of how to evaluate drugs in advanced prostatic cancer is reflected in the publication of Jones et al. [4] about objective response criteria in phase II and III studies in advanced prostatic cancer. Either one adopts the EORTC Genito-Urinary Group view that the only objective way to assess the efficacy of an investigational agent in advanced prostatic cancer is to use bi-dimensional by measurable soft tissue and visceral lesions, using WHO 1979 definitions of complete response (CR) and partial response (PR) only [5], *or* one adopts the view of the NPCP [6] which has adopted criteria which are much weaker and more difficult to assess, especially in bone. These result in a much higher response rate but are open to debate.

The more strict EORTC criteria are supported by Yagoda [7] and Tannock [8].

I have adopted a similar critical standpoint as that of the various authors of the chapters on genito-urinary regimens in successive volumes of the EORTC chemotherapy annuals [9-15].

The results of the chemotherapeutic trials of the NPCP have been presented by Elder and Gibbons [6] in sufficient detail to allow the analysis presented in Table 1. The patients in these studies had failed hormone therapy, had metastatic disease and were assessed according to the NPCP criteria of response. The 'stable disease' category used by the NPCP as an objective indicator of response is not generally accepted. If one examines the objective response rates of the patients shown in Table 1 only in respect of complete and partial responses, then none of the agents shown could be said to have any adequate activity.

Table 1. Summary of % responses seen in NPCP chemotherapy studies in advanced prostate cancer patients

Protocol	Drug(s)	No.pts.	Reported responses (%) CR	PR	Stable	Prog.	% excluded from analysis after randomisation
			Patients without extensive prior irradiation				
100	Cyclophosphamide	41	0	7	39	54	12
	5-FU	33	0	12	24	64	
	Standard treatment	36	0	0	19	81	
300	Cyclophosphamide	35	0	0	26	74	22
	DTIC	55	0	4	24	72	
	Procarbazine	39	0	0	13	87	
700	Cyclophosphamide	43	2	5	28	65	22
	Me-CCNU	27	0	4	26	70	
	Hydroxyurea	28	4	4	7	86	
1100	Methotrexate	58	2	3	36	59	16
	Cisplatin	50	0	4	32	64	
	Estramustine	50	0	2	32	66	
			Patients with extensive prior irradiation				
200	Estramustine	46	0	6	24	69	16
	Streptozotocin	38	0	0	32	68	
	Standard treatment*	21	0	0	19	81	
400	Estramustine + Prednimustine	54	0	2	11	87	14
	Prednimustine	62	0	0	13	87	
800	Estramustine	27	0	4	22	74	26
	Vincristine	34	0	3	12	85	
	Both drugs	29	0	0	24	76	
1200	Estramustine	40	0	0	18	82	17
	Cisplatin	42	0	0	21	79	
	Both drugs	42	0	0	33	61	

* Supportive care, radiotherapy, hormones etc.
(after Tannock IF, 1985)

Table 2. Apparently ineffective cytotoxic drugs in advanced prostate cancer objective (CR + PR) rates < 10%

BCNU	Hydroxyurea	Neocarzinostatin
Busulphan	M-AMSA	Peplomycin
CCNU	Methyl-CCNU	Procarbazine
Cyclophosphamide	Melphalan	Spirogermanium
DTIC	Methotrexate	Streptozotocin
Esorubicin	Mithroymycin	Vincristine
5-Fluorouracil	Mitoxantrone	VP16-213

After analysing the data of the EORTC chemotherapy annuals up to 1985 and the data presented by Carter and Wasserman [16], Braich et al. [17], Moore et al. [18], Dexeus et al. [19] and Scher et al. [20], one can conclude that the agents shown in Table 2 are ineffective under the conditions tested and with the response criteria utilised, since the objective response rate consisting of CR and PR only is less than 10%.

Activity is normally defined in cancer chemotherapy as an objective response rate (CR + PR) of more than 20%. Among cytotoxic drugs reported as active, doxorubicin has been found to have a response rate ranging from 15 to 25%. It must be mentioned that this holds both for 3-week high-dose doxorubicin and weekly low-dose (20 mg/m^2) treatment [21,22]. At lower doses the response rate dropped, as was reported by Robinson et al. [21]. The critical dose level of this drug family is also reflected in the recent EORTC study using epirubicin at a dose of 12 mg/m^2 weekly, which did not result in a useful objective response rate. Further studies with higher doses of this agent are suggested [23]. Both the vinca alkaloids vindesine and vinblastine give a response rate of approx. 20%. It must be mentioned, however, that vindesine 3 mg/m^2 weekly is rather neurotoxic in this elderly group of patients and that the quoted response rate for vinblastine has only been observed during 5-day continuous infusion therapy which in this older group of patients is not very palliative. In conclusion, the available data indicate that single-agent activity is essentially modest. The activity is also frequently associated with marked toxic effects, especially in patients with unfavourable prognostic features such as advanced age or advanced disease.

Mitomycin C has been tested recently in the EORTC group as a single-agent study with very strictly defined response criteria [24]. In 31 evaluable patients (of 37 entered), including 6 patients with no prior therapy for this cancer, a partial response was demonstrated in 9 patients. On the basis of this response rate mitomycin C is now being compared against estramustine phosphate in a randomised phase III study of the EORTC GU group for patients failing first-line hormonal treatment. It must be mentioned, however, that patients who obtain a partial response with mitomycin C in the dose of 10 to 15 mg/m^2 at 6 to 8-weekly intervals might develop renal toxicity above a cumulative dose level of 50 mg/m^2.

One of the problems so far not addressed is whether one should stop hormonal treatment when starting chemotherapy. From the literature no definite data can be derived. In my opinion patients enrolled in phase II studies (when the intention is to properly identify the response of the drug under study) should be taken off hormonal treatment. However, in general, when a drug with a proven activity is applied and the hormonal activity still might have a palliative effect in some of the disease sites, one is prepared to combine the 2 treatment modalities in the hope of achieving better palliation. There are no data in the literature, though, proving that the combination of hormonal therapy and chemotherapy results in a higher response rate in advanced prostatic cancer, nor are there any data supporting the application of combinations of cytotoxic drugs in patients with advanced prostatic cancer.

The final recommendations that can be made are the following:

1) In a patient with advanced metastatic prostatic cancer the first option is hormonal treatment. For the optimal selection of this primary hormonal treatment the reader is referred to previous chapters. The priority of hormonal treatment over chemotherapy is obvious to me as hormonal treatment results in a 40% objective response rate and always has less side effects than chemotherapy, thus giving better palliation.

2) The decision as to how to proceed after failure of hormonal treatment is not clear. An answer might come from the ongoing EORTC trial in which such patients are randomised between estramustine phosphate and mitomycin C.

Until these data are available my preference, if the patient is still in a good condition (reflected by a Karnofsky performance index of 100% or 90%, or WHO performance score of 0 or 1), would be to offer second-line hormonal treatment or to enroll the patient in a chemotherapy protocol. Patients who have measurable disease defined according to Jones et al. [24] should enroll in proper phase II studies to identify drugs (hormones or cytotoxic drugs) which may be more active against this disease.

REFERENCES

1 Kearsly J: Cytotoxic chemotherapy for common adult malignancies: "The emperor's new clothes" revisited? Br Med J 1986 (293):871-876
2 Murphy GP: Chemotherapy: is it effective in treatment of prostatic cancer? Urology 1984 (24 Suppl):41-47
3 Eisenberger MA, Simon R, O'Dwyer PJ, Wittes RE, Friedman MA: A re-evaluation of non-hormonal cytotoxic chemotherapy in the treatment of prostatic carcinoma. J Clin Oncol 1985 (3):827-841
4 Jones WG, Akaza H, Van Oosterom AT, Kotake T: Objective response criteria in phase II and phase III studies. In: Schröder FH et al (eds) Progress in Urological Oncology II. Alan R Liss, New York (in press)
5 WHO Handbook for Reporting Results of Cancer Treatment (1979). World Health Organisation. Offset Publication No 48, Geneva
6 Elder JS, Gibbons RP: Results of trials of the USA National Prostatic Cancer Project. In: Schröder FH, Richards B (eds) Therapeutic Principles in Metastatic Prostatic Cancer. Alan R Liss, New York 1985 pp 221-242
7 Yagoda A: Cytotoxic agents in prostate cancer: an enigma. Semin Urol 1983 (1):311-321
8 Tannock IF: Is there evidence that chemotherapy is of benefit to patients with carcinoma of the prostate? J Clin Oncol 1985 (3):1013-1021
9 Ozols RF, Yagoda A: Genito-urinary tumours. In:Pinedo HM, Chabner BA (eds) Cancer Chemotherapy /7 (The EORTC Cancer Chemotherapy Annual). Elsevier, Amsterdam/New York/Oxford 1985 pp 347-365
10 Stoter G, Rozencweig M, Pinedo HM: Genito-urinary tumours. In: Pinedo HM (ed) Cancer Chemotherapy 1979 (The EORTC Cancer Chemotherapy Annual 1). Excerpta Medica, Amsterdam/Oxford 1979 pp 317-339
11 Stoter G, Williams SD: Genito-urinary tumours. In:Pinedo HM, Chabner BA (eds) Cancer Chemotherapy 1983 (The EORTC Cancer Chemotherapy Annual 5). Elsevier, Amsterdam/New York/Oxford 1983 pp 357-368
12 Stoter G, Williams SD, Einhorn LH: Genito-urinary tumours. In: Pinedo HM (ed) Cancer Chemotherapy 1980 (The EORTC Cancer Chemotherapy Annual 2). Excerpta Medica, Amsterdam/Oxford 1980 pp 306-320
13 Stoter G, Williams SD, Einhorn LH: Genito-urinary tumours. In:Pinedo HM (ed) Cancer Chemotherapy 1981 (The EORTC Cancer Chemotherapy Annual 3). Excerpta Medica, Amsterdam/Oxford 1981 pp 317-332
14 Williams SD, Stoter G, Einhorn LH: Genito-urinary tumours. In:Pinedo HM (ed) Cancer Chemotherapy 1982 (The EORTC Cancer Chemotherapy Annual 4). Excerpta Medica, Amsterdam/Oxford 1982 pp 298-308
15 Williams SD, Stoter G: Genito-urinary tumours. In:Pinedo HM, Chabner BA (eds) Cancer Chemotherapy /6 (The EORTC Cancer Chemotherapy Annual). Elsevier, Amsterdam/New York/Oxford 1984 pp 344-362
16 Carter SK, Wasserman TH: The chemotherapy of urologic cancer. Cancer 1975 (36):729-747

17 Braich T, Ahmann FR, Garewal HS, Robertone A, Salmon SE: Phase II trial of 4'-deoxydoxorubicin (esorubicin) in hormone resistant prostate cancer. Invest New Drugs 1986 (4):193-196
18 Moore MR, Troner MB, De Simone P, Birch R, Irwin L: Phase II evaluation of weekly cisplatin in metastatic hormone-resistant prostate cancer: a South-Eastern Study Group trial. Cancer Treat Rep 1986 (70):541-542
19 Dexeus FH, Logothetis C, Samuels ML, Hossan B: Phase II study of spirogermanium in metastatic prostate cancer. Cancer Treat Rep 1986 (70):1129-1130
20 Scher HI, Sternberg C, Heston WDW, Watson RC, Niedzwiecki D, Smart T, Hollander P, Yagoda A: Etoposide in prostatic cancer: experimental studies and phase II trial in patients with bidimensionally measurable disease. Cancer Chemother Pharmacol 1986 (18):24-26
21 Robinson MRG, Chandrysekran S, Newling DWW, Richards B, Smith PH: Low dose doxorubicin in the management of advanced carcinoma of the prostate. Br J Urol 1983 (55):747-748
22 Torti FM, Aston D, Lum BL, Kohler M, Williams R, Spaulding JT, Shortliffe L, Freiha FS: Weekly doxorubicin in endocrine-refractory carcinoma of the prostate. J Clin Oncol 1983 (1):477-482
23 Jones WG, Fossa SD, Bono AV, Klijn JGM, De Pauw M, Sylvester R: An EORTC phase II study of low dose weekly epirubicin in metastatic prostate cancer (submitted for publication)
24 Jones WG, Fossa SD, Bono AV, Croles JJ, Stoter G, De Pauw M, Sylvester M: Mitomycin C in the treatment of metastatic prostate cancer: report of an EORTC phase II study. World J Urol 1986 (4):182-185

The Clinical and Financial Implications of Immediate or Deferred Treatment in Patients with Advanced Prostatic Cancer

Philip H. Smith

Department of Urology, St. James's University Hospital, Leeds, U.K.

Cancer of the prostate may be diagnosed because of symptoms of outflow obstruction, the effect of the local tumour on surrounding organs including the bladder (haematuria) and rectum (constipation or a feeling of fullness), by extension to the peritoneum producing discomfort, or by symptoms from metastases (occult cancer). It may come to light coincidentally following a prostatectomy for what was thought to have been benign disease (latent cancer) and is increasingly being diagnosed in Western Europe and the United States following routine health screening. Once diagnosed, the management will be determined by the stage of the disease and the therapeutic inclination of the surgeon.

Patients with disease localised to the prostate may be offered deferred treatment, radical prostatectomy or radiotherapy (externally or by interstitial techniques). Those with disease beyond the prostate are usually treated by hormonal manipulation, with or without radiotherapy to the local tumour or to painful metastases. After the failure of primary treatment, second-line hormonal therapy and cytotoxic chemotherapy may be used. As yet the cytotoxic agents have not shown sufficient promise to suggest that they are of any value at the time of initial treatment.

This contribution is devoted not to the continuing debate upon radical prostatectomy or radiotherapy for the patient with disease localised to the prostate, but to a consideration of the benefits and disadvantages of immediate and deferred treatment for the patient with disease beyond the prostatic capsule and for those with metastases. Some assessment is also made of the desirable frequency of follow up and of the likely cost of the different treatment options.

Choice of Treatment

Since the introduction of hormonal therapy by Huggins and Hodges in 1941 it has been possible to offer treatment with some hope of success to patients with metastatic prostatic cancer. Symptoms are relieved in 80% of those affected and objective response is seen in approx. 30% of patients [1,2]. Following the report of the Veterans Administration Cooperative Research Group (VACURG) in 1967 [3], which demonstrated the cardiotoxicity of stilboestrol 5 mg a day, a large variety of alternative compounds have become available including estramustine phosphate, progestogens (e.g. medroxyprogesterone acetate) and antiandrogens of the steroidal and non-steroidal types (e.g. cyproterone and flutamide).

The majority of these agents have now been studied in prospective randomised clinical trials, the new compounds being compared against conventional treatment. From the observations of Andersson et al. [4], Murphy et al. [5], Pavone-Macaluso et al. [1] and Smith et al. [2], it seems clear that cyproterone acetate, estramustine phosphate and medroxyprogesterone acetate have not been demonstrated to have any overall superiority over stilboestrol or orchidectomy in first-line treatment.

In 2 of these studies [1,2] a dose of stilboestrol 1 mg 3 times a day was used and De Voogt et al. [6] have recently demonstrated the cardio-toxicity of this dose of stilboestrol.

It is known that some patients take their tablets intermittently, since they demonstrate normal levels of testosterone at follow up and yet seem to remain in good health. As a result, some surgeons have come to consider the possibility of intermittent therapy [7] and also the possibility of deferring therapy until such time as it is required for obvious progression or for the relief of symptoms [8].

Timing of Therapy

The finding of cancer of the prostate clinically beyond the prostatic capsule or the discovery of metastases is an event of great significance for the individual patient who can readily appreciate that his tumour is unlikely to have been present at birth and that its discovery is associated with its progression. At this point, he becomes concerned about the possible rate of progression and the measures which can be taken to prevent it. This leads naturally to a philosophy of immediate treatment, using the agents which are known to be the most effective - in this instance orchidectomy or hormonal therapy.

Despite this simple logic, those who have been particularly interested in this disease are still uncertain whether immediate hormonal treatment in a patient without symptoms is of benefit in prolonging life or in prolonging the total symptom-free interval. Scott [9] stated "I am one of those who believe that hormonal treatment in prostatic cancer should be reserved for the patient who has metastases which are causing pain" and Cockburn [10] believes that "such treatment should be delayed until the onset of symptoms when its effect will be more readily appreciated by the patient."

Paulson found no benefit for radical radiotherapy in a trial comparing it and delayed androgen deprivation for patients with non-metastatic disease beyond the prostatic capsule. The time to first evidence of disease progression and survival was the same in both groups, suggesting that radiotherapy had not influenced the outcome [11]. In an earlier paper Paulson reviewed the concept of deferred therapy for patients with disease localised to the prostate and came to a similar conclusion when he stated that "multi-modal therapy consisting of pelvic lymphadenectomy with or without external beam radiotherapy has no benefit over surgery or no treatment" [12].

Newling et al. [13], Parker et al. [14] and Handley et al. [15] have investigated the outcome in patients in whom treatment has been deferred for one reason or another. In 130 patients reported by Newling et al. [13], 57 had disease beyond the prostatic capsule or had metastases. In a follow up extending from 6 to 141 months only 17 patients died of prostatic cancer with an average length of survival of 18.4 months. In a similar but non-randomised group of 130 treated patients there were 33 deaths from prostatic cancer in a follow up of 1 to 8 years (mean 4.3 years).

Parker et al. [14] carried out a retrospective survey of 263 patients with prostatic cancer with a minimum follow up of 5 years. Of these, 91 had demonstrable bone metastases at presentation, 115 were without metastases at presentation and in 35 patients the M category could not be classified. Of the 241 patients 173 received anti-cancer treatment at diagnosis whilst 68 did not. Of these 42 were category M0. There was no difference in time to first or second progression in the treated and untreated patients without metastases. In patients with demonstrable metastases hormonal manipulation hardly influenced the time to first progression and did not influence overall survival in the group of 79 treated and 12 untreated patients. Parker et al. concluded that delayed treatment is justified in prostatic cancer and noted that in their hands 36% of M0 patients needed no anti-cancer therapy within 5 years of diagnosis.

Handley et al. [15] reviewed 278 patients managed by deferred treatment after relief of bladder outflow obstruction. Within 3 years, treatment was required for progression in half the patients, the indication for therapy being local progression in 3 of every 4 patients. At the time of review the mean follow up was 41 months and 78% of patients had required treatment. The 37 patients with asymptomatic metastases at presentation were treated only when symptoms developed or progression occurred. Of these, 4 (11%) were alive and needed no treatment after 3 years of follow up.

From this information it does seem apparent that immediate therapy is not associated with an obvious reduction in mortality from cancer of the prostate. These observations, together with the conclusions of Paulson and Scott, emphasize the continuing uncertainty. Although the majority of the profession incline towards the view that clinical presentation implies progression and thus the need for treatment at the time of diagnosis, the arguments in favour of such a course of action (especially in patients with no symptoms) have never been conclusively proved. If anything, a critical and logical interpretation of previously published results including those from the Veterans Administration Cooperative Urological Research Group argue against immediate treatment unless for the relief of symptoms, a point recently highlighted by Fair [16]. Those who accept the concept that treatment is not immediately indicated in the absence of symptoms must then decide whether treatment is indicated upon progression or only when such progression is symptomatic.

If the treatment for this condition was curative, the argument for immediate therapy would be difficult to resist. However, the only effective treatment is palliative and although 80% of patients with symptoms do obtain symptomatic relief (and are thus to some extent hormone responsive), only 30% have an objective response [2]. Many patients do not have symptoms other than outflow obstruction at diagnosis and it is not known whether these patients have a greater, similar or lesser *total* symptom-free interval if hormonal therapy is given immediately in the absence of symptoms other than obstruction, which can of course be relieved by transurethral resection. The topic is of considerable interest as treatment has its drawbacks in terms of reduction of libido, impotence, and, in the case of female hormonal therapy, a tendency to cardiovascular complications.

Table 1. Average costs of out-patient and in-patient treatment at St. James's University Hospital, Leeds, for the year ended March 1986

Out-patient consultation:	New patient	£ 126.38
	Follow-up visit	24.99
In-patient costs:	Per day	74.74
	Average per case	724.67

Financial Implications of Immediate or Deferred Treatment

Management of the patient involves diagnosis, treatment and follow up and usually demands a period of time in hospital. In the United Kingdom most hospital costings are approximate. In a given hospital the overall cost of the out-patient and in-patient service can be determined. When these costs are divided by the number of patients attending or admitted, the average costs per attendance or per in-patient day can be established. These figures do not relate to the charges levied on private patients. The costs of out-patient and in-patient attendance at my own hospital are shown in Table 1.

Although the diagnostic procedures will be similar in all patients, the attitude to therapy will produce significant variations in overall costs because of the differing prices of the treatment options and the variations in frequency of follow up that may stem from these decisions (e.g. monthly visits for LHRH injections) or from a decision to defer treatment in the absence of symptoms.

Diagnosis

The essential aspect of diagnosis is histological proof of prostatic cancer. In addition, it is customary to carry out a full blood count, blood urea and electrolytes, acid and alkaline phosphatase, chest X-ray, IVP, bone scan and perhaps a plasma testosterone. The cost of these investigations in the United Kingdom is shown in Table 2.

Table 2. Approximate U.K. costs of basic diagnostic tests (1987)

Diagnostic test	Cost (£)
Needle biopsy	7.00
Full blood count	7.00
Blood urea and electrolytes	7.00
Plasma testosterone	7.00
Chest X-ray	5.00
Intravenous pyelogram	47.00
Bone scan	70.00
Total	150.00

Table 3. Annual costs of hormonal treatment (UK prices) 1987

Drugs	Cost (£)
DES 1 mg daily	7.54
Medroxyprogesterone acetate 100 mg bd	155.00
Cyproterone acetate 100 mg tds	1,084.00
LHRH analogue (Zoladex depot)	1,573.00
Orchidectomy (4-day stay)	300.00

Treatment

Most doctors are aware of the general issues considered in determining the choice of a given drug. However, many have yet to realise that not all products have the same or even similar costs.

The U.K. costs of the common forms of therapy are shown in Table 3. The cost of orchidectomy assumes a total in-patient stay of 4 days whilst the drug costs are those required to treat the patient for 1 year with the agent chosen.

It is immediately clear that DES is the cheapest form of therapy and that all options other than MPA exceed the cost of an orchidectomy within 1 year of initiation of therapy. The indications for the use of the alternative agents must, therefore, be based upon some factor other than financial outlay and must depend upon the conviction of the superiority of the form of treatment chosen. Such conviction is seldom backed by incontrovertible scientific evidence.

Follow Up

A few surgeons initiate treatment and ask that the patient be referred for further assessment only if problems arise, based upon the presumption that no alternative form of therapy is likely to be effective upon relapse and assuming that the patient or his doctor will have the wisdom to initiate a further referral upon the development of anaemia, uraemia or bone pain, all of which may respond to further treatment.

However, most prefer to follow their patients at intervals of 3 to 6 months, enquire about symptoms, carry out a full clinical examination, and check the haemoglobin, urea and phosphatases, carrying out bone scans every 6 to 12 months.

Clearly regular follow up is even more vital in monitoring those in whom treatment is being deferred because of a lack of symptoms. In such patients close clinical supervision and repeated investigation are required in order that treatment may be offered at the first sign of progression, especially of bone pain consistent with incipient pathological fracture, back ache giving rise to the possibility of spinal cord compression or uraemia.

For those on deferred therapy a 3-monthly visit is probably mandatory with clear information that the patient should re-attend earlier at the first sign of unexplained symptoms. In centres advocating a deferred treatment policy it is likely that the follow-up costs will be higher than in those in which treatment is initiated at the time of diagnosis. The true value of such an approach, however, will be determined not by the overall cost but by the benefit, if any, to the patient. This matter is now being addressed in certain clinical trials.

Trials of Immediate and Deferred Treatment

Prospective randomised clinical trials need to recruit large numbers of patients. It is easier to do this if 2 similar forms of therapy are being compared than if the options are obviously different, e.g. radical radiotherapy versus an operation. A trial which compares immediate or deferred therapy is even less likely to attract commitment despite the fact that the interest may be great and the answer of enormous importance for both quality of life and overall survival.

Disease Localised to the Prostate

Cancer localised to the prostate may be treated by radiotherapy or by radical surgery. The evidence from Paulson's study [11] is that radiotherapy is not superior to deferred treatment in patients whose disease has penetrated the prostatic capsule. For patients whose tumour lies within it there appear to be no published results of randomised trials comparing radiotherapy with deferred treatment or other forms of therapy. The Medical Research Council did recruit 75 patients to one such study but the results have not yet been published. The Urological Group of the EORTC (European Organisation for Research and Treatment of Cancer) considered a trial of immediate versus deferred radiotherapy in category T2-4 Nx M0 disease but this study has not been implemented.

The evidence from the randomised studies of radical prostatectomy versus placebo carried out by the Veterans Administration Cooperative Urological Research Group (VACURG) suggests that there is little difference in survival following radical operation or deferred therapy of patients within the first 10 years. Despite this, however, the progression rate was greater in the group not subject to radical operation and further analysis of the 111 patients in the 2 trials carried out by the VACURG may yet show differences which would be significant, at least for the younger patients with a life expectancy in excess of 10 years [17,18].

Disease beyond the Prostatic Capsule

The possibility of deferred hormonal therapy was first seriously considered after the inital report of the VACURG [3] who showed that placebo *as inital treatment* was not associated with impaired survival in patients with disease beyond the prostatic capsule and in those with metastases. In a subsequent study in much smaller numbers of patients (36 randomised to radical radiotherapy and 41 to delayed androgen ablation), Paulson showed no benefit for radiotherapy in patients with category T0-2 N+ M0 disease in terms of time to progression or survival. In a similar study of patients with category T3 N0 M0 disease, 40 patients were treated by radiotherapy and 33 received androgen ablation by orchidectomy or stilboestrol 1 mg tds when progression occurred. In this group also there was no difference in the time to first evidence of treatment failure or in survival up to 5 years.

At 5 years almost 60% (58% of each group) had no detectable evidence of progression [11,19]. These studies suggest that radical external beam radiotherapy is unlikely to be of benefit to the patient with non-metastatic but node-positive or extracapsular disease, except in so far as it may help in control of the primary lesion.

This conclusion is currently being tested again by an EORTC study (EORTC Protocol 30846, coordinator F. Schröder, Rotterdam) in which patients who are known to be node positive following lymph node dissection but who have no evidence of metastases (Tx pN1-3 M0) are randomised to receive immediate or delayed endocrine treatment at the time of progression (Fig. 1). The endocrine treatment chosen is depot LHRH (zoladex) 3.6 mg every 4 weeks and cyproterone acetate 50 mg tds in the hope of producing total androgen blockade. Patients randomised to deferred endocrine treatment will start therapy when objective progression is noted and may also be treated if non-specific (subjective) change occurs including significant deterioration of performance status, or marked increase in pain, acid phosphatase or alkaline phosphatase. This study is still recruiting and is not likely to be analysed for some time.

There appear to be no recent publications in which patients with asymptomatic disease have been offered the possibility of deferred treatment on a randomised basis. This lends increasing interest to the current study organised by the Urological Group of the Medical Research Council in which patients with disease clinically beyond the prostatic capsule who are non-metastatic patients or who have asymptomatic metastases (irrespective of the category of the primary tumour) are randomised to immediate or deferred orchidectomy [8].

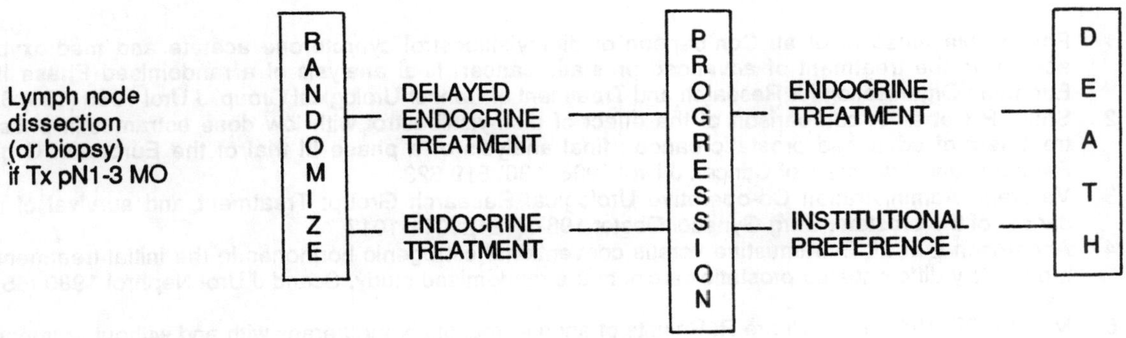

Fig. 1. EORTC protocol 30846. Immediate versus delayed endocrine treatment in Tx pN1-3, M0 disease after lymph node dissection (Coordinator F. Schröder, Rotterdam).

The importance of such a study has been emphasized both by Stamey [20] and by Fair [16]. Despite the difficulties inherent in such a trial, the coordinator, Mr. Kirk of Glasgow, has encouraged an entry in excess of 350 patients in a 2-year period. The analysis of the results must be delayed for some years but will be of great interest to all urologists. In this study patients are stratified between M0 and M1 at entry. The analysis will include total symptom-free survival, time to progression and overall survival as assessed using a simple annual enquiry form.

Conclusions

Despite enthusiasm for radical operation and radical radiotherapy for the patient with localised disease, and despite the introduction of the different estrogens, progestogens, anti-androgens, LHRH analogues and the concept of total androgen blockade for the patient with disease beyond the prostatic capsule, the correct management of prostatic cancer remains controversial.

The place of radical surgery for the patient with disease localised to the prostate has yet to be incontrovertibly established and recent evidence suggests that radical radiotherapy for the patient with extra-capsular disease offers little hope of controlling progression. No agent has yet been shown to be superior to stilboestrol 1 mg daily in relieving symptoms and in producing objective response.

It is recognised that therapy for prostatic cancer is usually palliative and there is increasing interest in determining whether treatment should be given at the time of diagnosis or may safely be deferred until progression of the disease is apparent. The current EORTC trial 30846 (coordinator Professor Schröder, Rotterdam) and the MRC trial of immediate and deferred orchidectomy (coordinator Mr. Kirk, Glasgow), should help to solve this basic question which carries with it clinical consequences of importance to every affected patient and financial consequences of interest to the community at large.

REFERENCES

1 Pavone-Macaluso M et al: Comparison of diethylstilbestrol cyproterone acetate and medroxyprogesterone acetate in the treatment of advanced prostatic cancer: final analysis of a randomised Phase III trial of the European Organisation for Research and Treatment of Cancer Urological Group. J Urol 1986 (136):624-631

2 Smith PH et al: A comparison of the effect of diethylstilbestrol with low dose estramustin phosphate in the treatment of advanced prostatic cancer: final analysis of a phase III trial of the European Organisation for Research and Treatment of Cancer. J Urol 1986 (136):619-623

3 Veterans Administration Co-operative Urological Research Group: Treatment and survival of patients with cancer of the prostate. Surg Gynecol Obstet 1967 (124):1011-1017

4 Andersson L et al: Estramustine versus conventional estrogenic hormones in the initial treatment of highly or moderately differentiated prostatic carcinoma: a randomised study. Scand J Urol Nephrol 1980 (55, Suppl):143-145

5 Murphy GP, Huben RP, Priore R: Results of another trial of chemotherapy with and without hormones in patients with newly diagnosed metastatic prostate cancer. Urology 1986 (28):36

6 De Voogt et al: Cardiovascular side effects of diethylstilbestrol, cyproterone acetate, medroxyprogesterone acetate and estramustine phosphate used for the treatment of advanced prostatic cancer: results from European Organisation for Research and Treatment of Cancer trials 30761 and 30762. J Urol 1986 (135/2):303-307

7 Klotz LH et al: Intermittent endocrine therapy for advanced prostate cancer. Cancer 1986 (58):2546-2550
8 Kirk D: Trials and tribulations in prostate cancer. Br J Urol 1987 (59):375-379
9 Scott WW: Panel discussion on some aspects of urological endocrinology. In: North Central Section of the American Urological Association Postgraduate Seminar. Burger, Minneapolis, p 211. Cited by Thompson GJ: Long term control of prostatic cancer. Surg Clin North Am 1958 (39):963-971
10 Cockburn AG: Hormonal therapy: the benefits of postponed initiation. Urology 1984 (24):24-26
11 Paulson DF, Hodge GB Jr, Hinshaw W, and the Uro-Oncology Research Group: Radiation therapy versus delayed androgen deprivation for stage C carcinoma of the prostate. J Urol 1984 (131):901-902
12 Paulson DF: Multi modal therapy of prostatic cancer. J Urol 1981 (17):53
13 Newling DWW et al: The natural history of prostatic cancer - the argument for a no treatment policy. In: Pavone-Macaluso M, Smith PH and Bagshaw MA (eds) Testicular Cancer and other tumors of the Genito-Urinary Tract. Alan R Liss, New York 1985 pp 443-448
14 Parker MC et al: Is delayed treatment justified in carcinoma of the prostate? Br J Urol 1985 (57):724-728
15 Handley RC et al: Deferred treatment for prostatic cancer. Br J Urol 1987 (in press)
16 Fair WR: Hormonal therapy of advanced prostatic cancer. J Urol 1986 (136):653-654
17 Byar DP: VACURG studies of post-prostatectomy survival. Scand J Urol Nephrol 1980 (55, Suppl):113-116
18 Byar DP: Review of the Veterans Administration Studies of cancer of the prostate and new results concerning treatment of stage I and II tumours. In: Pavone-Macaluso M, Smith PH and Edsmyr F (eds) Bladder Tumors and other Topics in Urological Oncology. Plenum, New York 1979 pp 471-492
19 Paulson DF: Treatment of locally confined prostatic cancer: radiotherapy versus surgery; limits of curability. In: Kurth KH, Debruyne FMJ, Schröder FJ, Splinter TAW and Wagener TDJ (eds) Progress and Controversies in Oncological Urology. Alan R Liss, New York 1984 pp 483-492
20 Stamey TA: Monographs in Urology 1985 (6):105

Treatment Recommendations for Daily Practice

S. Rocca-Rossetti

Department of Urology, University of Turin, Turin, Italy

Prostatic cancer is the second or third cause of cancer morbidity in elderly males in Europe and is of major interest in daily urological practice. About one in every 100 males can be expected to develop a clinically detectable cancer of the prostate during his lifetime. The ageing of the European male population will increase the absolute number and incidence. The problem is complicated by the fact that over 90% of the patients with prostatic cancer present with advanced disease at the time of diagnosis and must be treated as having incurable disease. Great efforts are being made in studies concerning the prevention, screening and early diagnosis of this tumour where loco-regional therapy may lead to a cure or to a remission that will last for the natural life of the patient. Here the presence of focal carcinoma, present in over 50% of patients over 70 years of age, poses another problem - that of therapy or surveillance. This Monograph deals with the medical treatment of advanced prostatic cancer and the previous chapters have covered some basic considerations and clinical overviews of the many possible therapeutic options available to the physician in his routine practice. The proliferation of new agents, the differing drug categories and the option of single or combined treatment has opened a Pandora's box in which many conflicting reports reflect the therapeutic enigma of advanced prostatic cancer, caused by the "natural" history and clinical evolution of the disease. Among the many prognostic factors that will define the outcome are the age and vital status of the patient, all the subjective and objective evidence of disease, the differentiation and metastatic behaviour of the tumour and the toxicity of the treatment given.

Diagnosis

The first duty of the physician is to diagnose the extent of the disease and to evaluate it in its clinical context in the life of the patient. TNM classification of tumours of the prostate (ICD 0 185) uses the symbols T, N and M, where T represents the primary tumour, N the regional lymph nodes and M the distant metastases.

The patient commonly seen presents with symptoms of dysuria and/or pain due to bone metastases. The clinical suspicion has to be confirmed by histological diagnosis, usually by needle biopsy of the primary tumour.

The histopathological diagnosis, by consideration of the tumour differentiation, will give an indication of the likely response to therapy. Though most tumours are multifocal and practically all are heterogeneous, one could state in broad general terms that well-differentiated prostatic cancer cells, closely resembling the normal acinar pattern, tend to respond much better to androgen withdrawal than cells of the anaplastic type.

Table 1. The TNM classification of tumours of the prostate

T_0	No evidence of tumour
T_1	Incidental histological finding
T_2	Limited to the gland
T_3	Invades apex, prostatic capsule, bladder neck, seminal vesicle, but is not fixed
T_4	Fixed or invasion of other structures
N_0	No regional lymph node metastases
N_1	Metastatic lymph node single 2 cm or less
N_2	Metastatic lymph node single between 2 and 5 cm in dimension, or multiple smaller metastases
N_3	Metastatic lymph node greater than 5 cm
M_0	No distant metastases
M_1	Distant metastases (further specification is possible)

A complete physical examination (in which the supraclavicular nodes should not be forgotten), a set of biochemical markers - prostatic acid phosphatase and alkaline phosphatase, and the routine haematological and biochemical data, followed by ultrasound imaging of the primary tumour, urography, chest X-ray and bone scan will give an indication of tumour extent. We recommend a graphic recording of the digital rectal examination for future comparisons. Computed tomography, bipedal lymphangiography and pelvic lymphadenectomy are essential only in those patients in whom distant metastases are not confirmed and in whom radical surgical excision is contemplated. Metastases are usually found in the bones (spine, pelvis, femora and rib) and are usually of the osteoblastic type. The visceral and soft tissue metastases (nodal masses, lung, liver) are predominant in 5 to 10% of the cases and have a worse prognosis.

Once the relevant data are available, the tumour should be classified according to the clinical TNM extent: T0-4, N0-3, M0-2 and G1-4, as shown in Table 1, which represents the relevant data from the 4th edition of the UICC booklet of the TNM system [1]. This edition is quite different from its predecessors since it involves clinical and pathological evaluations.

Treatment

It is widely accepted that patients with T3 disease, and all patients with N1-3 or M1 disease, are not suitable for loco-regional treatment, such as surgery and/or radiotherapy to the primary tumour and its regional lymph nodes.

The primary tumour sometimes progresses to bladder outlet obstruction and hydronephrosis where palliative transurethral resection is indicated to relieve urine retention. However, in some cases the treatment response to androgen withdrawal may be sufficient to decrease primary tumour volume and restore bladder function.

Despite the heterogeneous nature of these tumours, androgen withdrawal results in objective response in 50% of the patients, whilst subjective response occurs in approximately 80% of previously untreated patients. It is then obvious that first-line systemic treatment, if indicated by all the diagnostic evaluation, should consist of some type of androgen deprivation.

Although endocrine therapy has been advocated and sporadically practised since 1895, without discriminating between cancer and benign hyperplasia, the scientific base for orchiectomy or estrogen therapy in prostate cancer was established by Huggins and Hodges less than 50 years ago [2].

It was generally accepted that the clinical choice between diethylstilbestrol (DES) 5 mg a day and bilateral orchiectomy depended largely on patient preference, until the Veterans Cooperative Urological Research Group (VACURG) established the cardio-vascular side effects of DES [3].

More recently, anti-androgens, gonadotropin releasing hormone agonists and drugs blocking the release of adrenal androgens have promised fewer side effects and greater patient compliance, stimulating renewed therapeutic interest in the medical treatment of prostatic cancer.

The list of the most commonly used medication is presented in Table 2. Bilateral orchiectomy is added to the list as it is in widespread use in daily clinical practice.

Of all the newer alternative treatments for prostatic cancer discussed in the previous chapters, none has proved superior to bilateral orchiectomy or DES treatment in terms of objective response rates. The fear of surgical castration and the accelerated death rate from cardio-vascular complications from estrogen therapy may lead to a choice of medical castration by LHRH agonists or to anti-androgen treatment. This latter therapy may preserve potency in some instances, but fails in long-term use.

The simple conclusion is that no single drug treatment has been proven to be superior to bilateral orchiectomy and the best treatment option is based on the patient's preference, the safety of the medication and the cost of treatment [4]. One must then ask whether any combination of agents is superior to monotherapy in patients with

Table 2. First-line endocrine treatment

1. Bilateral orchiectomy
2. Interference with the hypothalamo-pituitary-gonadal axis
   - Estrogens
   - Luteinizing hormone releasing hormone agonists
   - Progestagens
3. Anti-androgens
   - Steroid and pure anti-androgens
4. Adrenal androgen steroid blockers

newly diagnosed prostatic cancer. Despite the impressive results for efficacy and safety reported by Labrie, who combined LHRH agonists and anti-androgens [5], no hard data have yet confirmed his hypothesis that combination treatment is superior because of its near total elimination of the adrenal androgens (see chapter 7). Labrie's data has come from phase II studies designed to quantify the activity of a treatment by objective evaluation of response in patients with measurable disease and have been compared with the results of historical series and of other randomized phase III trials. However, several large-scale randomized studies are now under way to help answering this question.

Evaluation of Treatment

The efficacy of hormonal treatment of advanced prostate cancer is still a matter of controversy, although new drugs and associations of drugs are being tested in clinical trials all over the world. The results of these trials are the subject of controversy for reasons related to the natural history and clinical evolution of prostate cancer, since

1. the disease has its highest incidence in men over the age of 70 and often presents a slowly progressive course;
2. crude survival data are sometimes misleading because death is frequently caused by concomitant diseases;
3. measurable metastases in lungs, liver, superficial lymph nodes and soft tissues are restricted to 5-6% of all patients and bone metastases are very difficult to quantify, even by bone scan;
4. only a moderate correlation has been found between reduction of prostatic acid phosphatase and response to treatment;
5. digital examination of the rectum to evaluate the primary tumour does not allow objective comparisons (though transrectal ultrasound is a reliable means of evaluating prostate mass);
6. the value of CT scan in the follow up of patients remains to be determined because of the incidence of false positive as well as false negative results;
7. the reduction of bone pain and urinary symptoms, generally achieved soon after the beginning of therapy, is common to every kind of treatment and might be influenced by other factors.

To evaluate the results of new therapies correctly, a standardization of response parameters, as indicated by the EORTC GU Group for phase II and phase III clinical studies, is necessary (some of these factors are shown in Table 3). A comparison of different treatments is possible only if patients are randomised in the treatment and control groups; so-called "historical" controls are of little value because of possible differences in the selection of patients. Most studies in prostatic cancer deal with time to progression and calculate response rates divided into complete and partial response, no change or stable disease, and progression. The most widely utilised response criteria are those developed by the NPCP and the EORTC [6,7]; the criteria listed in Table 3 were utilised in the EORTC studies [8]. However, as very few patients have measurable disease [9], the endpoints of the randomised studies are restricted to evidence of clear progression of disease or death from cancer. More recently, extra protocol studies on bone scans, markers, quality of life, pathology, endocrinology and response evaluation have been incorporated in the EORTC studies (EORTC protocols

Table 3. Response criteria in prostatic cancer

Measurable	Evaluable	
Lymph nodes	Primary tumour	Performance status
Subcutaneous deposits	Hot spots on bone scan	Pain
Nodular lung metastases	Ureteric dilation	Weight
Nodular liver metastases	Bone metastases on X-ray	Haemoglobin
	PAP (prostatic acid phosphatase)	Liver function tests
	PSA (prostate specific antigen	Phase reactant proteins
	GSM (gamma semino protein)	
Objective	Subjective	

30853-30864). The lesson to be remembered is that few reported studies provide all the data for proper evaluation and that only randomised studies can demonstrate treatment superiority if properly evaluated in a substantial number of patients.

At this moment there is no evidence that combination treatment aimed at blocking the possible hormonal influence of the adrenal androgens on prostatic cancer is of clinical benefit, when compared to single-drug therapy or surgical castration. Essentially all untreated patients that responded to the first-line hormonal therapy relapse by progressing to a state where the primary tumour and/or metastases are irresponsive to further androgen withdrawal treatment, no matter how aggressive the secondary treatment may be.

Second-line hormonal treatment seems effective only if the first-line treatment fails to bring the testosterone down to castrate levels [10]. However, some reports claim responses - mainly subjective - by the use of high doses of stilphostrol, progestins, adrenal inhibitors or anti-androgens (see chapter 5).

Unfortunately, the cell lines active at this stage of the disease are androgen independent and other treatments are indicated. One of those favoured is estramustine phosphate, a combination of hormonal and chemotherapy, in high doses. From the available literature we may conclude that estramustine phosphate, mitomycin C and doxorubicin seem to be effective agents with a 20 to 30% objective response and pain relief in up to 50% of the cases. Chemotherapy is, of course, of value only for a limited duration and we need to remember that the patient usually wants pain relief, which in appropriate cases can also be obtained by local irradiation of selected metastatic sites. The last question concerns the time at which active endocrine treatment should start. There is experimental evidence that early treatment prolongs the duration of the remission [11], but no randomised studies have yet proved this to be really the case in the clinical situation. Common sense dictates that pain, deterioration due to tumour and widespread disease should be treated early, while minimal invasive disease without symptoms deserves consideration for active surveillance.

In general, we may conclude that the newer endocrine treatments are only refinements of the classical treatment leading to surgical or medical castration. If one selects the alternative treatment, one should monitor the patient, know all the side effects and consider the cost of therapy. A constant surveillance of the literature with a critical evaluation of the reported results will protect the patient from the side effects of unestablished treatments. If the clinician follows the beaten path of established treatment, he will provide optimal "available" therapy for the patient in daily practice. All alternative treatment should first be carefully evaluated in clinical trials where the safety of the patient is safeguarded by constant monitoring.

REFERENCES

1 Hermanek P, Sobin LH (eds) TNM Classification of Malignant Tumours, 4th edition. Springer Verlag, Berlin 1987

2 Huggins C, Hodges CV: Studies of prostatic cancer. Effect of castration, estrogen and androgen injection on serum phosphatase in metastatic carcinoma of the prostate. Cancer Res 1941 (1):293-297

3 Veterans Administrative Cooperative Urological Research Group: Treatment and survival of patients with cancer of the prostate. Surg Gynecol Obstet 1967 (124):1011-1017

4 Robinson MRG, Hetherington J: The EORTC studies: is there an optimal endocrine management for M1 prostatic cancer? World J Urol 1986 (4):171-175

5 Labrie F, Dupont A, Belanger A: Complete androgen blockade for the treatment of prostatic cancer. In: De Vita VT, Hellman S, Rosenberg SA (eds) Important Advances in Oncology. Lippincott Comp, Philadelphia 1985 pp 193-217

6 Murphy GP, Slack NH and participants in the National Prostatic Cancer Project: Current status of the National Prostatic Cancer Project treatment protocols. In: Denis L, Murphy GP, Prout GR, Schröder F (eds) Controlled Clinical Trials in Urologic Oncology. Raven Press, New York 1984 pp 119-133

7 Smith PH, Pavone-Macaluso M, Viggiano G, De Voogt H, Lardennois B, Robinson MRG, Richards B, Glashan RW, De Pauw M, Sylvester R and the EORTC Urological Group: EORTC protocols in prostatic cancer. In: Denis L, Murphy GP, Prout GR, Schröder F (eds) Controlled Clinical Trials in Urologic Oncology. Raven Press, New York 1984 pp 107-117

8 Newling DWW: Criteria for response to treatment of metastatic prostatic cancer. In: Schröder FH, Richards B (eds) Therapeutic Principles in Metastatic Prostatic Cancer. AR Liss Inc, New York 1985 pp 205-220

9 Jones WG: EORTC Phase II chemotherapy studies in prostate cancer. In: Schröder FH, Richards B (eds) Therapeutic Principles in Metastatic Prostatic Cancer. AR Liss Inc, New York 1985 pp 435-445

10 Keuppens F, Fossa S, Nowé P, Denis L: Secondary orchiectomy in patients with prostatic cancer in relapse. In: Denis L, Murphy GP, Prout GR, Schröder F (eds) Controlled Clinical Trials in Urologic Oncology. Raven Press, New York 1984 pp 207-209

11 Benson MC, Coffey DS: New concepts and controversies concerning prostate cancer. In: Kurth KH, Debruyne FMJ, Schröder FH, Splinter TAW, Wagener TDJ (eds) Progress and Controversies in Oncological Urology. AR Liss Inc, New York 1984 pp 547-562

U. Veronesi, B. Arnesjö, I. Burn, L. Denis, F. Mazzeo (Eds.)

European Handbook of Surgical Oncology

The Present State of the Art in Europe

1988. Approx. 80 figures. Approx. 1000 printed pages. ISBN 3-540-17770-1

The European Society of Surgical Oncology wishes to announce the imminent publication of the European Handbook of Surgical Oncology.

The first of its kind in Europe, this handbook will be an essential feature of every surgeon's library. It is a basic guide of the surgical approach to cancer treatment with contributions by the most prestigious names in oncology in Europe.

This handbook will be a MUST in years to come, an invaluable reference for all those with a specific interest in the field of oncology.

Springer-Verlag
Berlin Heidelberg NewYork
London Paris Tokyo

Springer

Already available:

F. Cavalli (Ed.)

Endocrine Therapy of Breast Cancer

1986. VII, 120 pages. ISBN 3-540-16959-8

J. F. Smyth (Ed.)

Interferons in Oncology

Current Status and Future Directions

1987. 70 pages. ISBN 3-540-18019-2

F. Cavalli (Ed.)

Endocrine Treatment of Breast Cancer II: Current Developments and New Methodologies

with the collaboration of: K. Brunner (Bern), R. Gelber (Boston), A. Goldhirsch (Bern), C. Jordan (Madison), H. Mouridsen (Copenhagen), S. Saez (Lyon)

1987. 8 figures. VII, 65 pages. ISBN 3-540-18339-6

L. Domellöf, Örebro, Sweden (Ed.)

Drug Delivery in Cancer Treatment

with the collaboration of: C. Van Groeningen (Amsterdam), S. P. Israels (Amsterdam), K. Lundholm (Göteborg), L. Paalzow (Uppsala), V. Ventafridda (Milan), P. Workman (Cambridge)

1987. ISBN 3-540-18459-7

The following title is in preparation:

H. M. Pinedo, Amsterdam; **M. J. Peckham,** London; **P. Winograd,** Amsterdam (Eds.)

Human Tumor Xenografts in Anticancer Drug Development

with the collaboration of: F. R. Balkwill (London), H. E. Blythman (Montpellier), E. Boven, (Amsterdam), B. J. M. Braakhuis (Amsterdam), J. Carmichael (Edinburgh), J. Fergusson (Edinburgh), H. H. Fiebig (Freiburg), O. Fodstad (Oslo), B. W. Fox (Manchester), F. Guiliani (Milan), L. R. Kelland (Surrey), P. Köpf-Maier (Ulm/Donau), J. Mattern (Heidelberg), S. Merry (Glasgow), R. Osieka (Essen), M. V. Pimm (Nottingham), J. Rygaard (Copenhagen), R. W. Shoemaker (Bethesda), J. F. Smyth (Edinburgh), G. G. Steel (Surrey), R. W. Bladwin (Nottingham)

Springer-Verlag
Berlin Heidelberg NewYork
London Paris Tokyo

Springer

MIX
Papier aus verantwortungsvollen Quellen
Paper from responsible sources
FSC® C105338

If you have any concerns about our products,
you can contact us on
ProductSafety@springernature.com

In case Publisher is established outside the EU,
the EU authorized representative is:
Springer Nature Customer Service Center GmbH
Europaplatz 3, 69115 Heidelberg, Germany

Printed by Libri Plureos GmbH
in Hamburg, Germany